Healthy Smoothie Recipes Book for Beginners

Easy Mix-and-Match Smoothie Recipes for a Healthier You

Camilla Leonard

Table of contents:

Introduction 6
Rules of the Perfect Smoothie 7
What You Need to Know About the Ingredients of the Perfect Smoothie 10
How to replace the ingredients in the recipe so that the smoothie remains perfect? 11
How to Make a Nut Milk 13
Smoothies for a Hearty Breakfast 16

    Blueberry, Orange and Dates Smoothie 16
    Morning Oats Smoothie 18
    Goji & Raspberries Smoothie 20
    Green Milk with Avocado 22
    Rich Chocolate Peach Smoothie 24
    Papaya Pineapple Smoothie 26
    Oatmeal Blueberry Smoothie 28
    Banana Almond Smoothie 30
    Cherry Cheesecake Smoothie 32
    Creamy Date Smoothie 34
    Dried Fruits Smoothies 36
    Raspberry Date Smoothie 38
    Cranberry-Banana Smoothie 40
    Banana Orange Protein Smoothie 42
    Mango Basil Smoothie 44
    Minty Mango Smoothie 46

Blueberry, Coconut & Peanut Butter Smoothie 48
Almond Smoothie Berry 50
Protein Smoothie 52

Smoothie Bowls 54
Protein Power Smoothie Bowl 54
Acai Breakfast Bowl 56
Berry Yogurt Smoothie Bowl 58
Chocolate Almond Smoothie Bowl 60
Chocolate smoothie bowl with coconut 62
Berry Smoothie Bowl 64
Green Smoothie Bowl 66
Green Smoothie Bowl with Peanut butter 68
Blue Smoothie Bowl 70

Diner 72
Healthy Brain smoothies 72
Berry Protein Shake 74
Protein Smoothie 76
Simple Protein Smoothie 78
Simple green smoothie 80
Full Protein Smoothie 82
Low-Sugar Smoothie 84
Cauliflower Smoothie 86
Green Coconut Smoothie 88
Banana Raspberry Smoothie 90

Green Detox 92
Celery and Beet Juice 92

Green Almond Milk Smoothie 94
Green Citrus Juice 96
Cold Fighting Green Smoothie 98
Fruit and vegetable cocktail 100
Kiwi Mint Smoothie 102
Avocado Smoothie 104
Green Lemonade 106
Sweet Spinach Detox 108
Celery Blueberry Smoothie 110

Warming Drinks 112
Spiced Apple Drink 112
Poached Pear Smoothie 114
Gingerbread Cookie Smoothie 116
Cold Fighting Green Smoothie 118

Summer Refreshing Smoothies 120
The Hydration Smoothie 120
Refreshing Coconut Lime Smoothie 122
Green Tea Juice 124
Refreshing Watermelon Juice 126

Introduction

Fruits and vegetables are naturally loaded with various kinds of nutrients which help people to keep healthy.

There are various purposes to add smoothies into your diet like it has anti-aging properties, healthy skin, meal replacement, weight loss, diabetes control, disease prevention and increases cognitive functions. Many fruits and vegetables include a wide range of antioxidants which helps to fight against many diseases provides heart disease and cancer. While you mix fruits and vegetables, you will surprise how well the taste of the smoothie. Smoothie is a concoction of juice, pulp, and skin of fruits and vegetables blending in a mixer. It's like a drink that is relatively smooth and requires little chewing. The smoothies in this book are specifically designed to be not only healthy and delicious but also excitingly energizing.

Enjoy!

Rules of the Perfect Smoothie

The main advice to make a perfect smoothie is to Experiment, but don't try to combine incompatible. Add different herbs and spices, nuts and grains, clavicle and muesli, chocolate and coffee. Some people like to add raw eggs. A great addition to a breakfast smoothie is oats. If you like dairy try to use milk, kefir, cottage cheese and yogurt. Vegetarians for the alternative could use fruit or vegetable juices, almond and rice milk or tofu. Everything that your heart desires...

- Don't add too much water; otherwise, instead of a thick cocktail, you will get liquid jelly. In order to get a rich taste and color, the consistency of the smoothie should be thick.

- Homogeneous texture — is the greatest success. In order for smoothies to be really tasty, it is important to get either a powerful blender or patience. In a green smoothie, you won't be able to find pieces of greens, dates and dried apricot mixed together with water create a creamy texture. Right, Smoothie looks like yogurt or milkshake; otherwise, you will get salad mixed with.

- Don't mix dark greens with berries. If you would like to mix spinach with strawberry, be prepared to get swamp water instead of pretty smoothly. It will be very difficult to make your friends try your concoction. Mask greens in you berry smoothie will be possible with dark color berries-blackberry, blueberry, currant.

- Add Nut Milk instead of Cow's Milk. Mixing fruits, berries or greens with Cow's Milk you got very heavy for digestion combinations, that doesn't bring benefits to your body. To get the right taste and constants for the milkshake, you will need the help of nut milk, which much better combines with fruits and greens. Make your own nut milk is super easy-you would need a blender, raw almonds, hazelnut or cashews.

- Sweetness- is the main ingredient of any smoothie. The most common of the sweet ingredients -is bananas. They add sweetness and creamy texture, also good mix with any berries and greens. Avocado can add a creamy texture too, but to sweeten it up you would need honey or maple syrup. In the chocolate shake with cocoa, you can add dates or dried apricot. Pears and mangos will be a great addition too.

- To avoid the too sugary taste, I always add the juice of lemon or lime.

- Know when to stop. Experiments are very interesting and fascinating, but some complicated combination could lead you to a disaster.

- Generally, perfect smoothie consists of 5 ingredients.
  For example: almond milk + spinach + banana + cherry;
  Or: almond milk + spinach + celery + banana. It is enough to find your favorite combinations and make them.

- Cold, but not icy. Never in my life, I met people who would prefer warm smoothies over cold ones. If your blender warms up the consistency while mixing, add cold water, not a room temperature one. Frozen berries also add some cold. I also like to add frozen bananas (Peeled, cut and frozen in the freezer)- shake is getting thicker, almost like frozen yogurt .

Professional blenders mix frozen berries with water very fast, so the drink doesn't get very cold. Other ones do it slower, and then we have a frozen shake. Too cold of the food doesn't digest easily by our body, so make sure you give it time to get a little warmer before you consume it.

What You Need to Know About the Ingredients of the Perfect Smoothie

Get the blues	Great greens	Wonderful white	Mellow yellow (and orange)	See red
Memory, healthy aging, urinary tract health	Vision, strong bones and teeth	Maintain healthy heart, cholesterol	Heart, vision, and immune system	Heart health, memory, urinary tract health
Fruits	**Fruits**	**Fruits**	**Fruits**	**Fruits**
Blackberries	Green apples	Brown pears	Apricots	Cherries
Blueberries	Green grapes	White nectarines	Cantaloupe	Red apples
Dried plums	Green pears	White peaches	Nectarines	Red grapes
Pitted prunes	Honeydew		Peaches	Red pears
Purple grapes		**Vegetables**	Yellow apples	Raspberries
Plums	**Vegetables**	Cauliflower	Yellow pears	Strawberries
	Asparagus	Garlic	Yellow watermelon	Watermelon
Vegetables	Broccoli	Kohlrabi		
Eggplant	Brussels sprouts	Onions	**Vegetables**	**Vegetables**
Purple asparagus	Chinese cabbage	Potatoes	Butternut squash	Beets
Purple cabbage	Cucumbers	(white fleshed)	Carrots	Radishes
Purple carrots	Green beans	White corn	Sweet corn	Red peppers
Purple peppers	Green cabbage		Sweet potatoes	Red onions
Potatoes	Green onions		Yellow beets	Rhubarb
(purple fleshed)	Green peppers		Yellow peppers	Tomatoes
	Leafy greens		Yellow potatoes	
	Lettuce		Yellow summer squash	
	Peas		Yellow tomatoes	
	Snow peas			
	Sugar snap peas			
	Zucchini			

How to replace the ingredients in the recipe so that the smoothie remains perfect?

When it comes to turning a full-fledged dish into a smoothie, it is important that there are vegetables in the smoothie, some fruit for sweetness and taste, healthy fats and proteins; basically, everything you find in food. This helps to ensure not only satiety but also that it is well balanced.

Variety of combinations are endless, and results are amazing.

Want to make the perfect smoothie, but don't have all the right ingredients? No problem! Here is a chart of the products that could be replaced by other ones. Now nothing can stop you from enjoying perfect smoothies.

Pineapple	Orange, grapefruit, mango, pear, banana, apple
Watermelon	Red grapefruit, cantaloupe, honeydew, tomato
Cucumber	Celery, zucchini, jicama
Lemon	Lime, grapefruit
Berries	Any type of fruit
Cashews + water	Coconut milk
Honey	Rice malt, maple syrup, condensed milk, dates
Banana	Plantain, avocado, pineapple
Blueberries	Strawberries, raspberries, blackberries, acai

Papaya	Pawpaw, strawberries
Coconut milk	Almond milk, coconut water, rice milk or any other preferred non-dairy milk
Almond butter	Any nut butter
Almond milk	Other dairy alternatives
Date	Honey or maple syrup
Orange	Mandarin, apple, pear
Ruby grapefruit	Yellow grapefruit
Ginger	Turmeric
Cherry	Berries
Green tea	Peppermint tea, white tea, fennel tea
1 scoop plant-based protein powder	3 tbsp hemp seeds
Mandarin	Orange, tangelo, carrots
Lime	Lemon, grapefruit
Celery	Zucchini, celeriac root
Kale	Lettuce, chard, spinach
Pears	Apple
Almond milk	Coconut milk, rice milk or any other preferred non-dairy milk
Dates	1 tsp of honey, maple syrup, stevia
Banana	Avocado; mango; frozen zucchini
Carrots	Parsnips
Chia seeds	Ground flaxseeds
Raspberries	Strawberries, blueberries

How to Make a Nut Milk

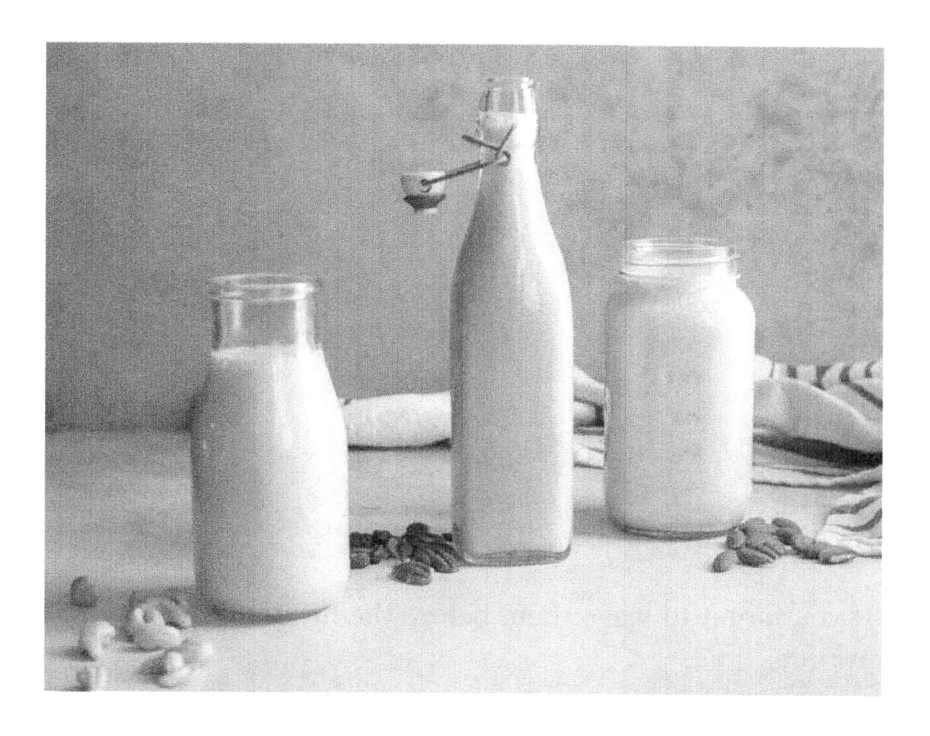

In our fridge, you always can find Nut Milk. With its help, any smoothie becomes tastier and more fulfilling. Nut Milk -Is a great alternative to regular milk, and to make one you don't need neither farm nor cows.

For Nut Milk, you would need water and any type of raw nuts. The tastiest milk you can get out of almonds, hazelnut, and Brazilian Nut. Some people use walnuts, Pine nuts and also you can make milk out of seeds- sesame, poppy or pumpkin.

Milk will be tastier if you soak the nuts for at least 4 hours in water beforehand. If you are making milk in the morning, leave the nuts in the bowl overnight. In the morning rinse and mix in the blender with a certain amount of water.

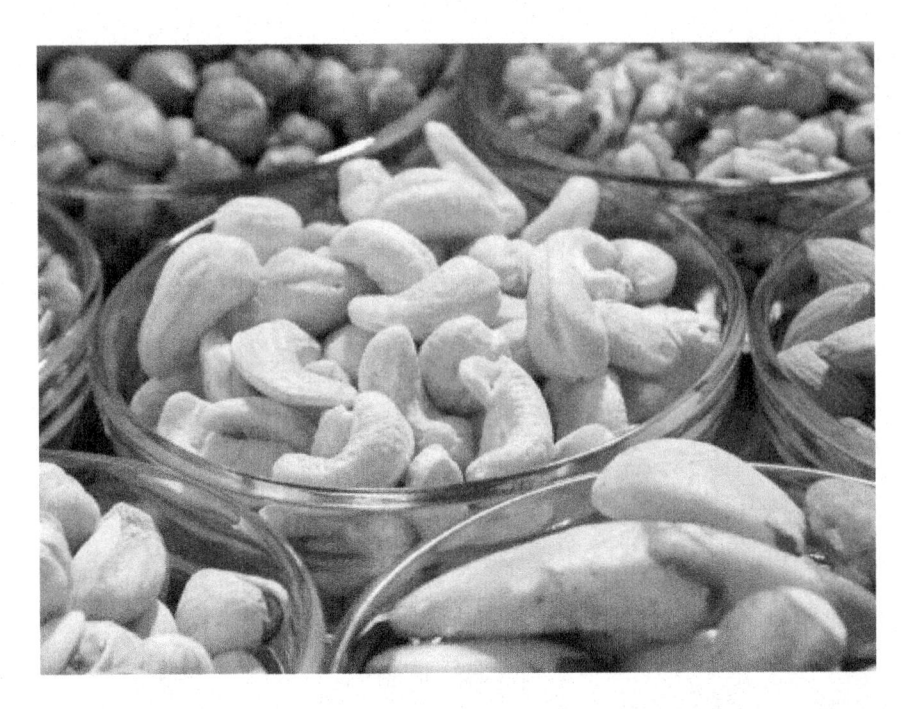

If you forgot to leave them before the head, no worries, just add dry, raw nuts.

Water-Almond Ratio:

There are so many different recipes for almond milk, some people swear by only adding 3 cups of water, while others religiously add 5 cups. This is an easy variable to play with, for thicker texture you can use less water. Personally, I tend to lean towards 4 cups.

Here is the Formula for the nut milk:

Nuts + Water+ Blender + sieve

Ingredients:

* For 4 cups of milk, you need 4 cups of water and 1 cup of nuts.
For 1 glass of milk: 1 cup of water and 1/4 cups of nuts.

Instructions:

1. Place nuts and water in a blender. You will see how simple water will become milk, while blender does its job. A more powerful blender will achieve homogeneous liquid faster.
2. Turn off the blender, pour through nut-milk bag or cheesecloth into a clean container.

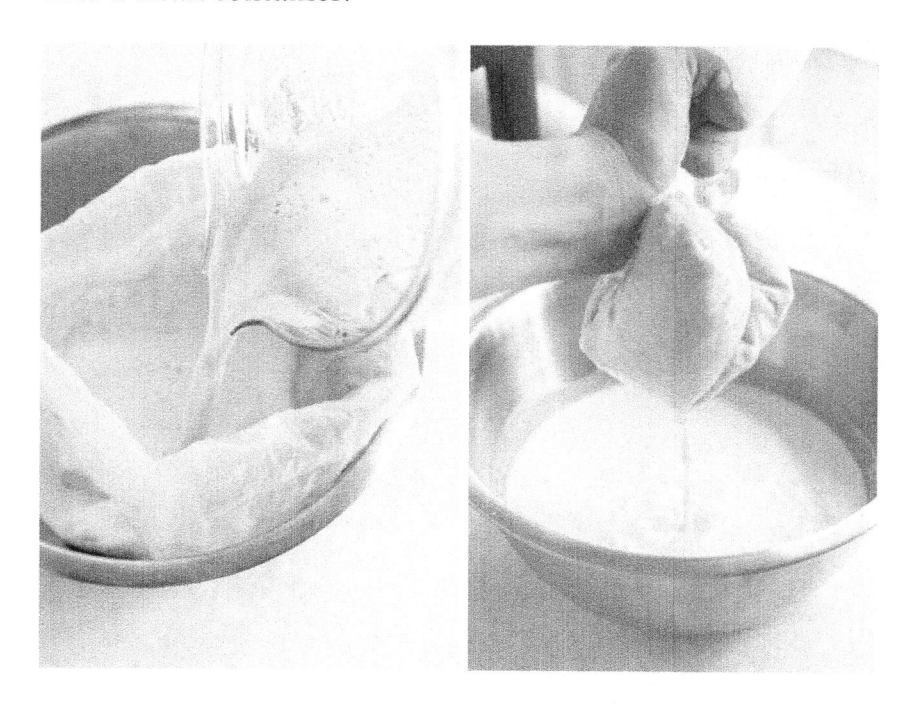

Keep refrigerated in a closed bottle around 3 days.

Smoothies for a Hearty Breakfast

No one loves to leave home hungry. But sometimes life happens, and you don't have time, to bake or cook anything. Sometimes you don't want to eat anything, and it takes so much energy to start your day. Then here comes a delicious smoothie to save your mood, to fill up your belly and your heart!

Blueberry, Orange and Dates Smoothie

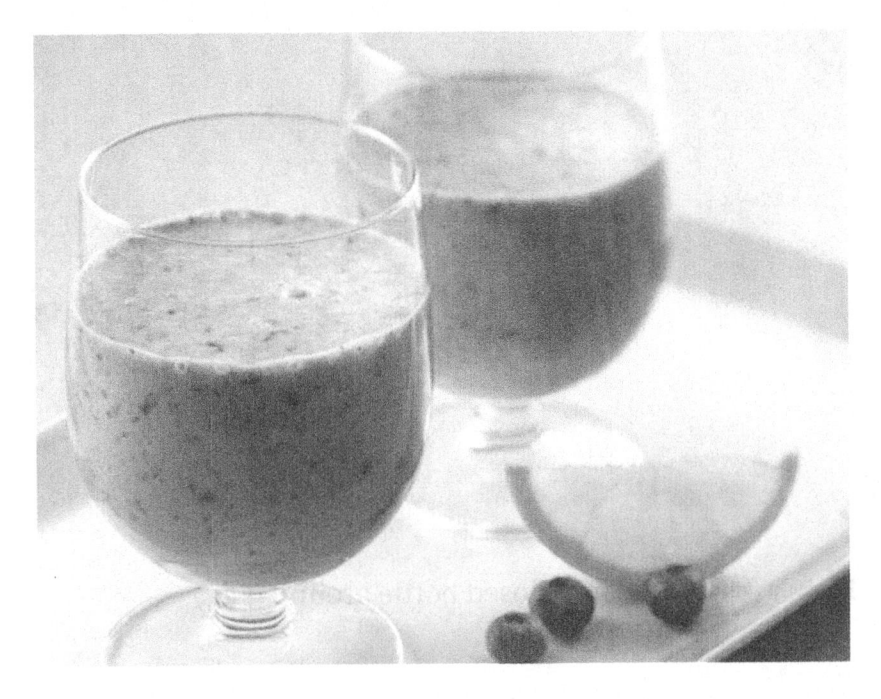

Ingredients:

- 100 g of frozen blueberries
- 25 g of dates
- 1 orange
- 14 g of walnuts

Instructions:

Place in blender frozen berries, dates without seeds and walnuts. Add an orange pulp and mix everything together.

Prep Time: 5 min

Serves: 2

Morning Oats Smoothie

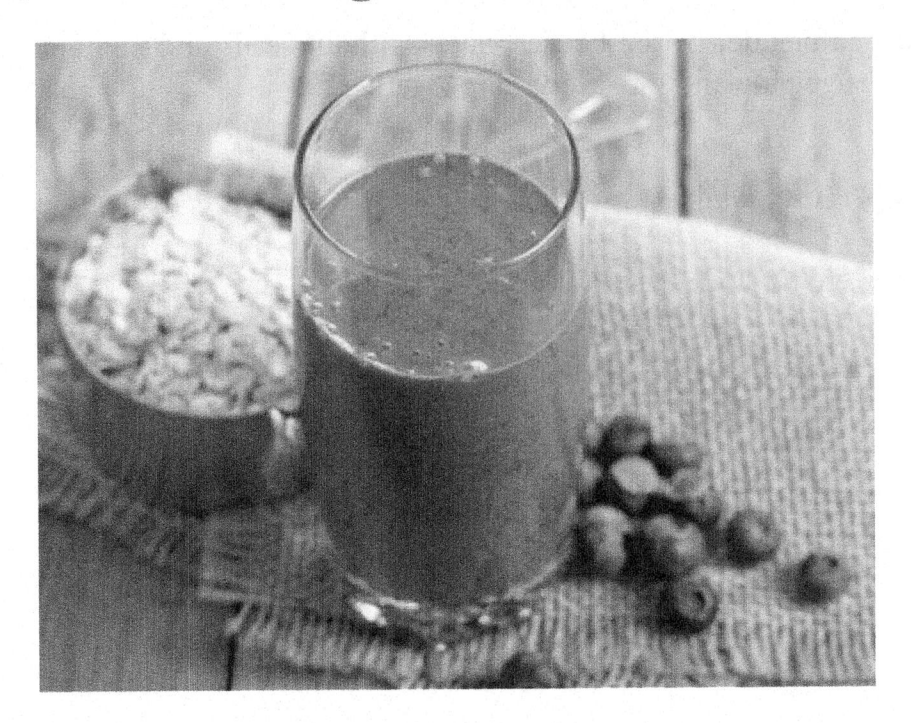

Ingredients:

- 1/4 cup (50g) rolled oats
- 1 banana, peeled and halved
- 1/2 cup (75g) blueberries
- 1 cup (250ml) coconut or almond milk (or whatever you like)
- 1 tablespoon maple syrup
- 1/2 teaspoon cinnamon
- Optional: 1 scoop protein powder

Instructions:

Add all ingredients into a high-powered blender and blend on high for at least 60 seconds until smooth.

Prep Time: 5 minutes

Servings: 1

Goji & Raspberries Smoothie

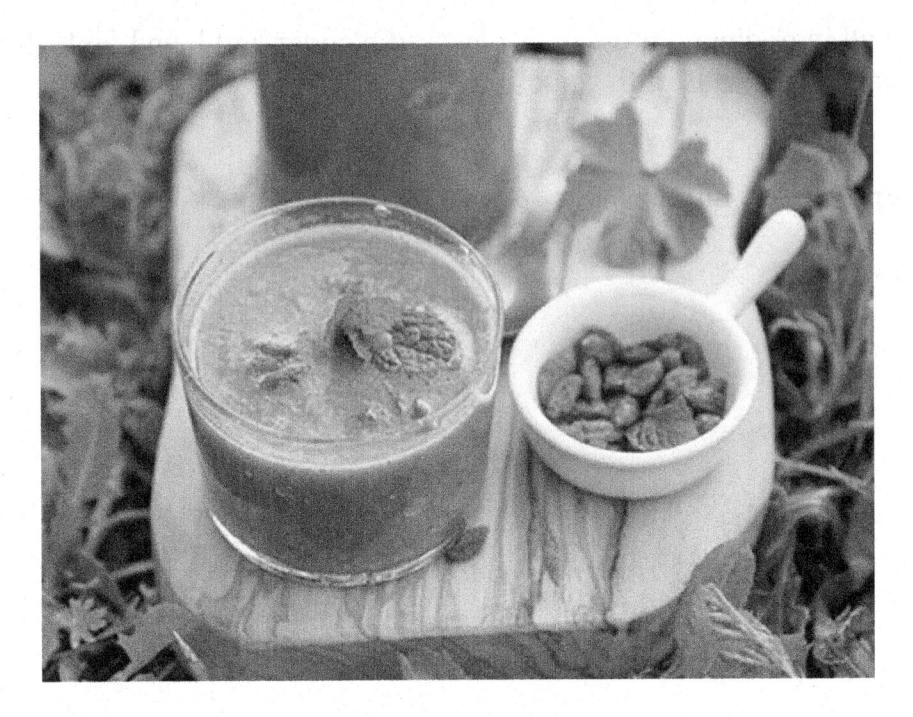

Ingredients:

- 2 Tbsp cashew butter
- 8-10 oz almond or hemp milk
- 3/4 cup frozen raspberries
- 1 Tbsp goji berries
- 1 tsp vanilla extract
- Dash of turmeric
- ½ cup ice

Instructions:

1. Wash and prepare the ingredients.
2. Combine all of the ingredients in a blender or food processor.
3. Blend or combine on high until well mixed, about 45-60 seconds.
4. Serve and enjoy!

Prep Time: 5 minutes

Servings: 1

Green Milk with Avocado

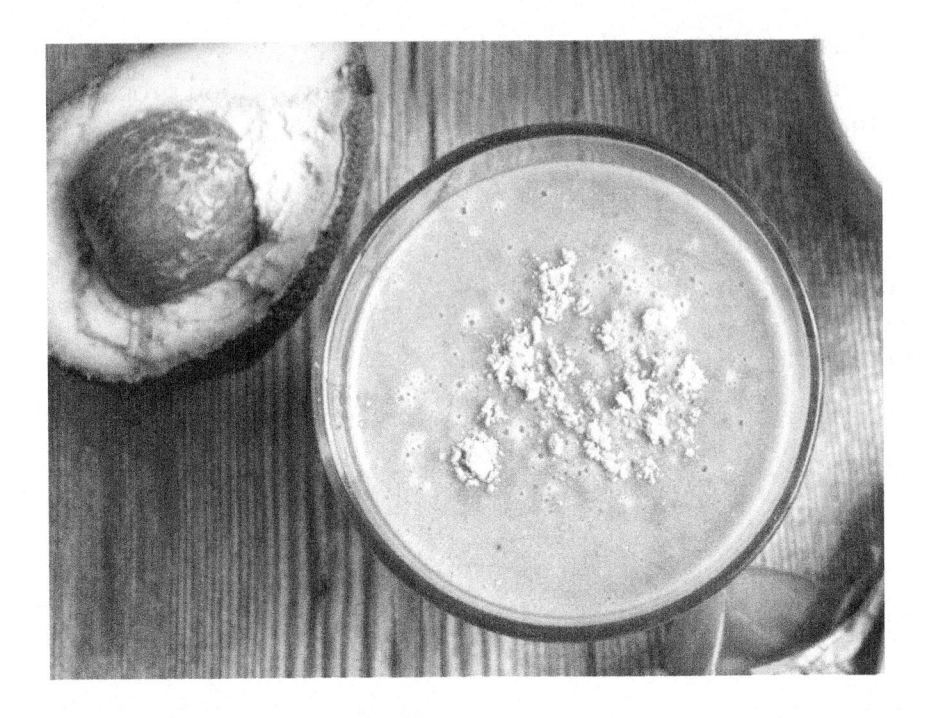

Ingredients:

- 1,5 cup of almond milk
- 100g of fresh spinach
- 1/2 avocado
- 1 teaspoon of honey or maple syrup
- 1 pinch of salt

Instructions:

1. Blend everything together. Your Green Milk is ready!
2. You can drink it by itself or add strawberries, peaches or other seasonal fruits.

Prep Time: 5 minutes

Servings: 1

Rich Chocolate Peach Smoothie

You're craving a satisfying treat, but you want to keep your health in mind? Chocolatey fruity smoothie includes nutrients that support heart and brain health due to the greens and healthy fat.

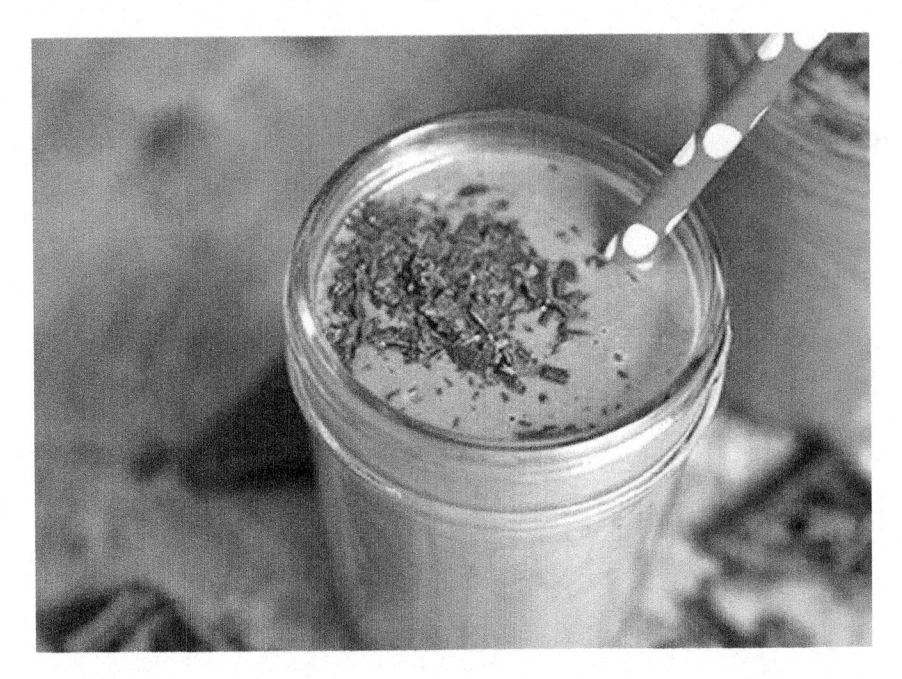

Ingredients:

- 1/2 cup (75 g) blueberries
- 1 peach
- 1/3 banana
- 1 handful of spinach or any greens
- 8 almonds
- 2 tbsp cacao powder
- 1 cup (250 ml) unsweetened almond milk

Instructions:

1. Wash all produce well.
2. Add ingredients through a blender and blend on high for 45-60 seconds until smooth.
3. Enjoy this sweet treat!
4. If you want the consistency to be thicker, you can add either 1/3 avocado or 1/2 banana, and if you want the smoothie slightly sweeter, you can also add one date.

Prep Time: 5 minutes

Servings: 1

Papaya Pineapple Smoothie

Delicious tropical smoothie for breakfast or as a snack. This smoothie is full of antioxidant compounds and fiber.

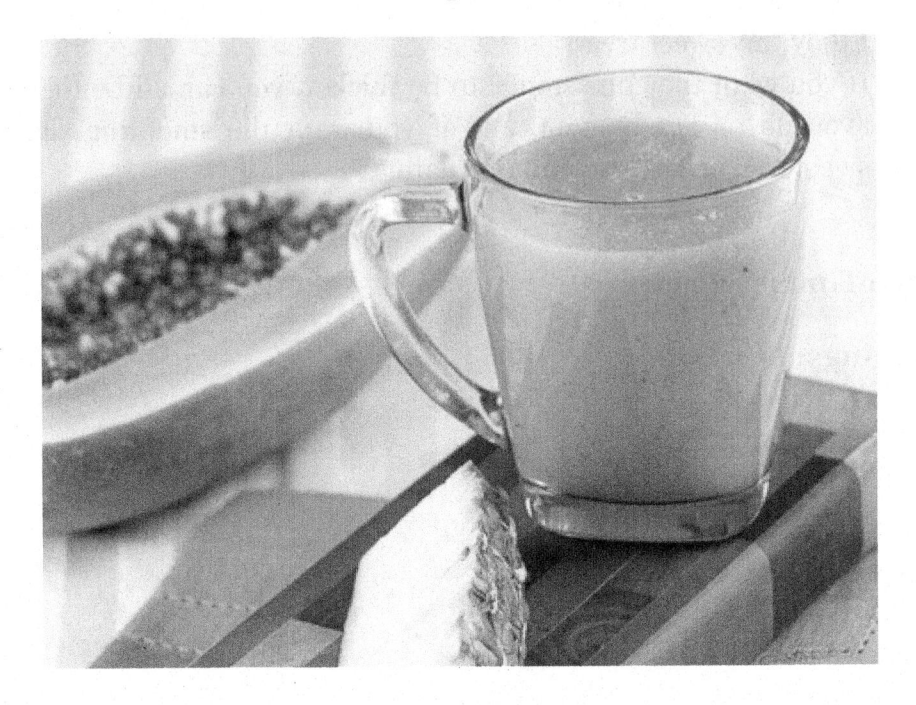

Ingredients:

- 1/8th of a fresh or frozen pineapple
- 1 frozen banana
- ¼ fresh papaya
- ½ cup of ice
- ½ cup of coconut milk
- 1 Tbsp of shredded coconut
- 2 tsp of chia seeds

Instructions:

1. Peel and chop the pineapple, banana, and papaya.
2. Add all the ingredients into the blender.
3. Blend & enjoy!

Prep Time: 10 minutes

Servings: 1

Oatmeal Blueberry Smoothie

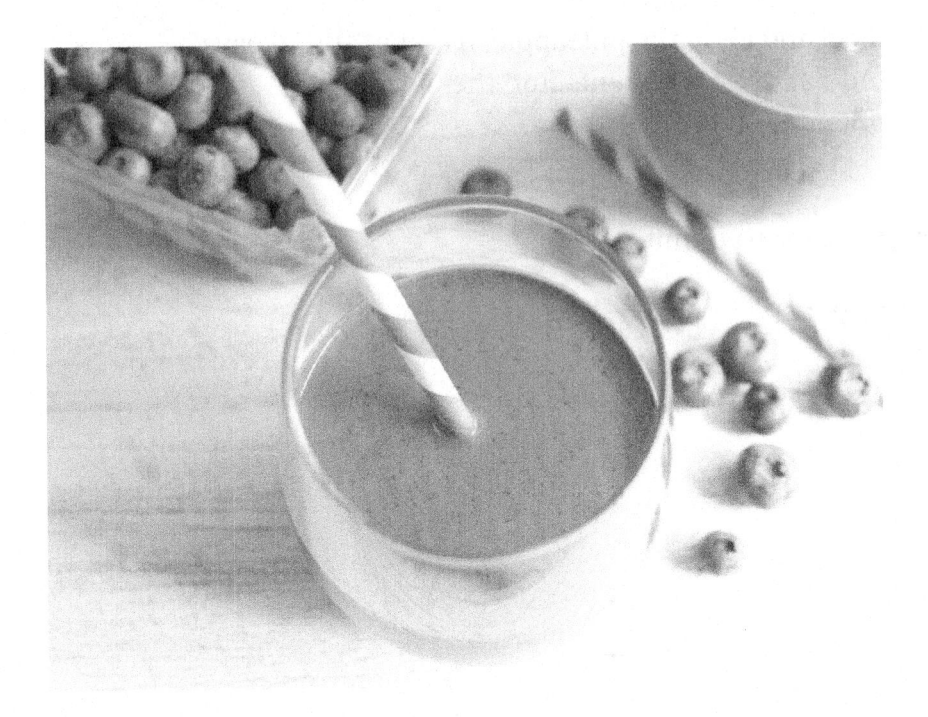

Ingredients:

- 1/2 cup of yogurt
- 1/2 cup of frozen blueberries
- 1/2 cups of rolled oats
- 2 ice cubes
- 1 teaspoon of honey
- 1/4 teaspoon of ginger

Instructions:

1. Place oats in the bowl add a little water and let it soak for 15 minutes.
2. All the ingredients and mix in the blender until smooth and creamy.
3. A nutritional smoothie is ready!

Prep Time: 5 min

Serves: 2

Banana Almond Smoothie

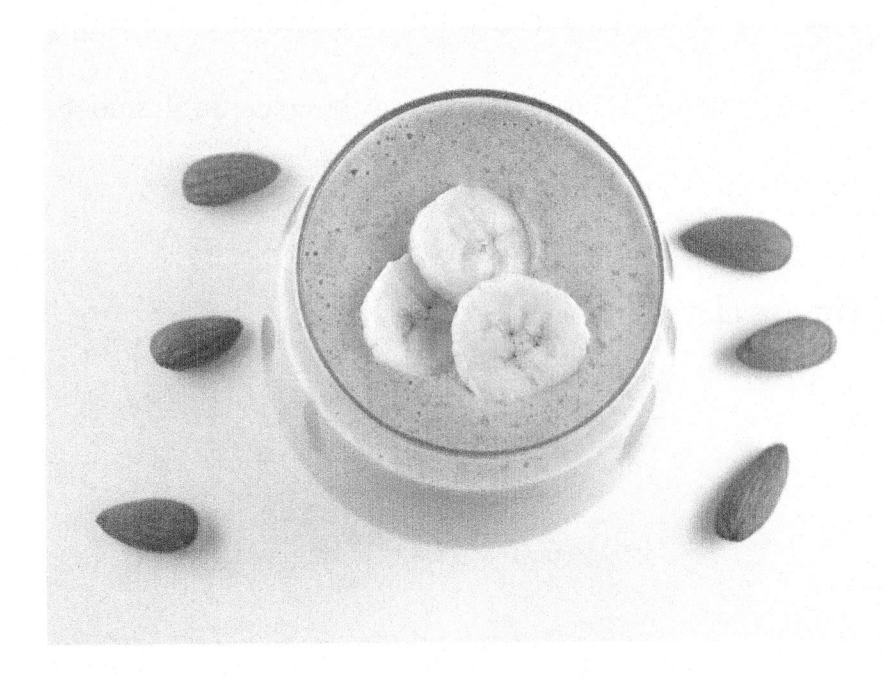

Ingredients:

- 1 banana
- 1/2 cup of plain yogurt
- 2 tablespoons rolled oats
- 10 almonds.
- 1 tablespoon of honey

Instructions:

1. Place everything in the blender and pulse until finely ground. The end result has to be smooth.
2. Enjoy!

Prep Time: 5 min

Serves: 2

Cherry Cheesecake Smoothie

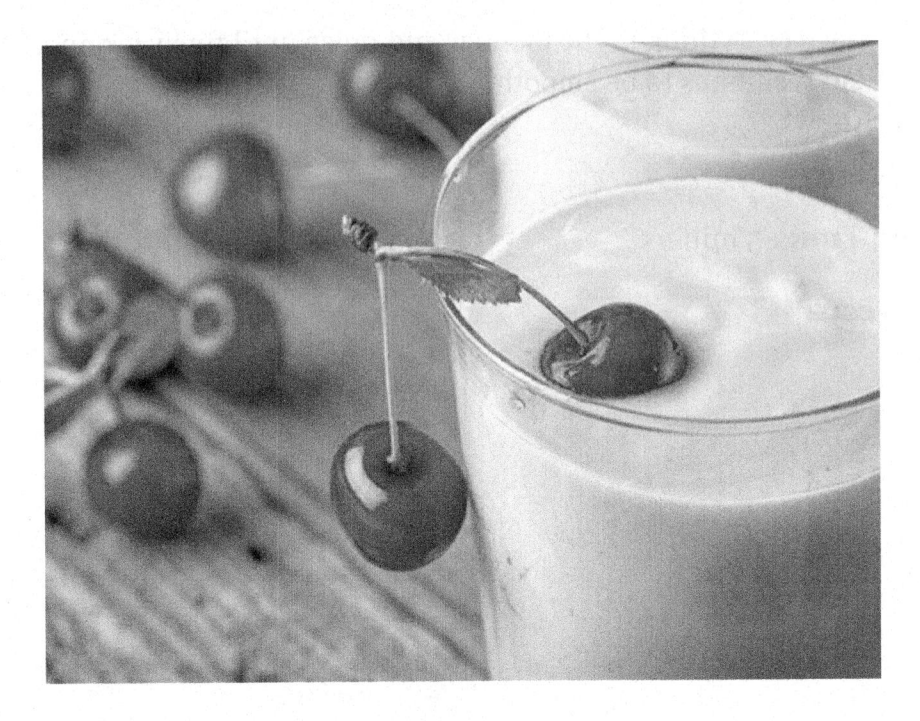

Ingredients:

- 1/2 cup of cheese or yogurt
- 1/2 cup of frozen cherry
- 1 banana
- 1 teaspoon of honey

Instructions:

Simply place all the ingredients and mix them until smooth and creamy.

Prep Time: 5 min

Serves: 2

Creamy Date Smoothie

Dates fiber-rich and contains nutrients such as potassium, calcium, and copper, which contribute to the health of your cardiovascular system.

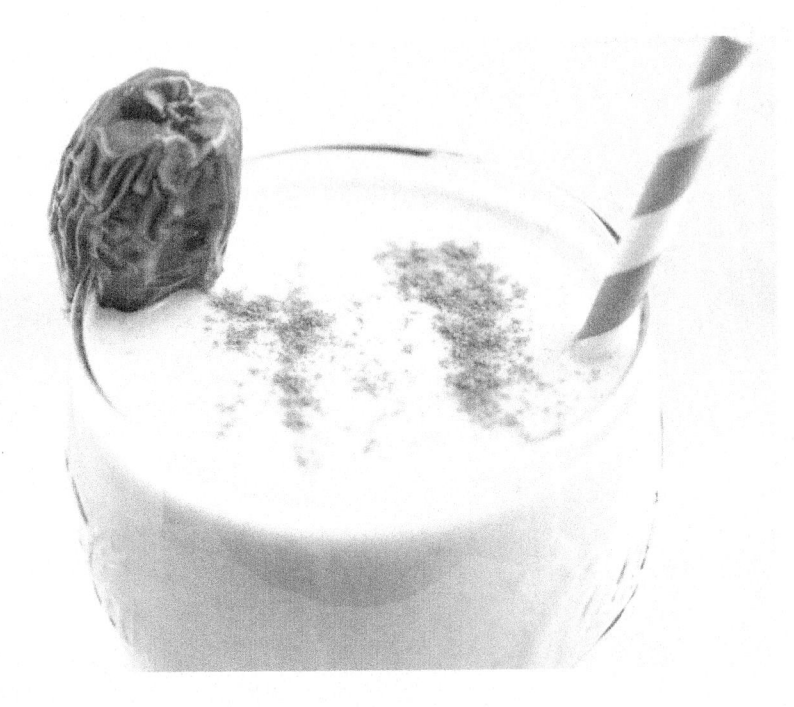

Ingredients:

- 2/3 cups of milk
- 1/3 cups of dates
- 2-3 ice cubes

Instructions:

1. Cut dates in half, if there are seeds inside, remove them, add milk and mix it in the blender.
2. Place the liquid in the fridge for 15 minutes, so the dates got softer.
3. After that add ice cubes and pulse until creamy.

Prep Time: 15 min

Serves: 2

Dried Fruits Smoothies

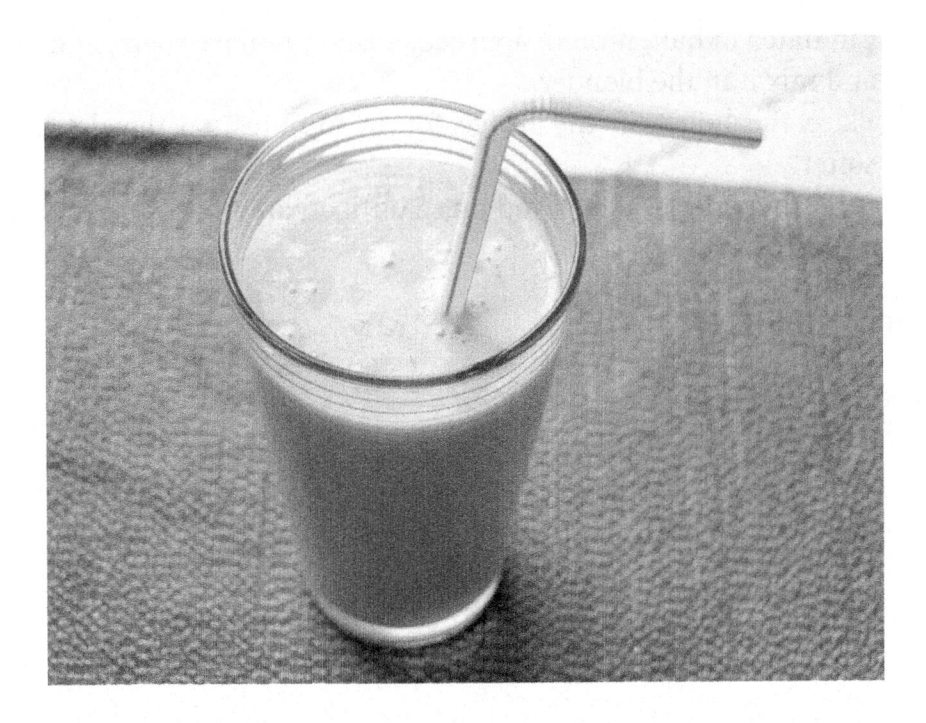

Ingredients:

- 1cup of Almond milk
- 1 tablespoon of rolled oats
- 1/4 cup of dried apricots
- 1/4 cup of dark raisins
- 1 tablespoon of honey

Instructions:

1. Wash dried fruits and pour boiling water. When they are softer, mix all the ingredients together.
2. Put the finished product in the fridge for 15 minutes to cool. After that, beat in a blender.
3. You can soak the dried fruits overnight in cold water, and in the morning make a smoothie for 3 minutes.

Prep Time: 15 min

Serves: 2

Raspberry Date Smoothie

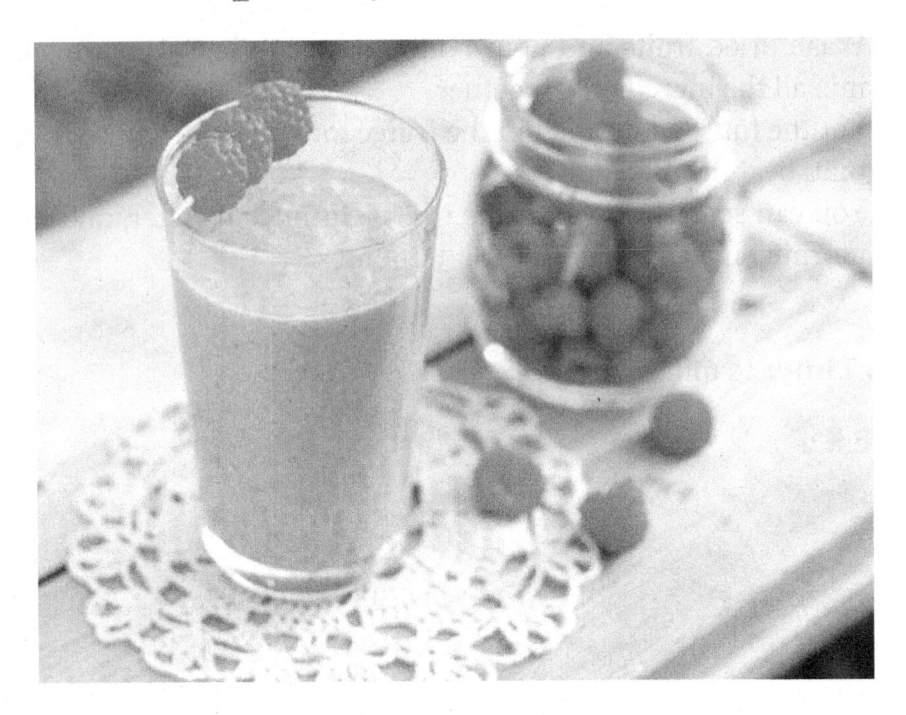

Ingredients:

Vanilla Layer
- ½ cup of almond milk
- 1 medjool date
- ½ tsp vanilla extract
- ½ cup of ice
- 1 tbsp. of white chia seeds

Raspberry Layer
- ¼ cup of almond milk
- 1 medjool date
- 1 cup of frozen raspberries
- 1 tbsp. of white chia seeds

Instructions:

1. Blend the vanilla layer ingredients and pour into a serving glass, store in the freezer while you make the raspberry layer.
2. Blend the raspberry layer ingredients and pour into the serving glass over the vanilla layer, then store in the freezer until ready to serve. Make sure you only chill not freeze the smoothie.
3. You can swirl the 2 layers with a straw and serve immediately.

Prep Time: 10 min

Serves: 1

Cranberry-Banana Smoothie

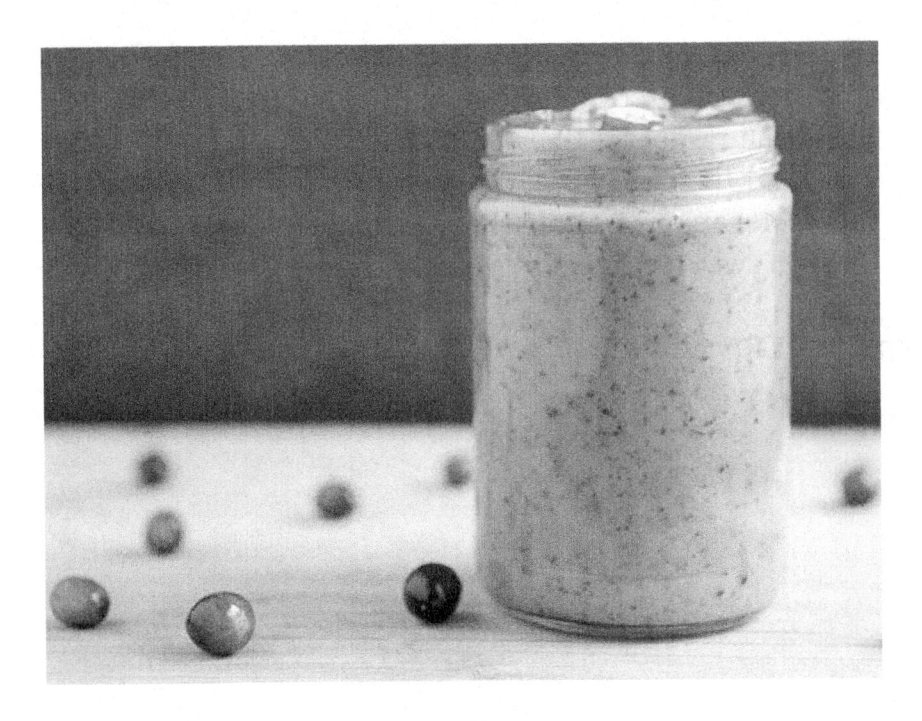

Ingredients:

- 200 ml of Kefir
- 1 banana
- 55 g dried cranberries
- 1 tablespoon of Flax Seeds
- 2 tablespoons of rolled oats
- 1 tablespoon of honey

Instructions:

1. Flaxseed, dried cranberries, and oatmeal pour warm for 15 minutes.
2. Blend everything together, until smooth and creamy.

Prep Time: 5 min

Serves: 2

Banana Orange Protein Smoothie

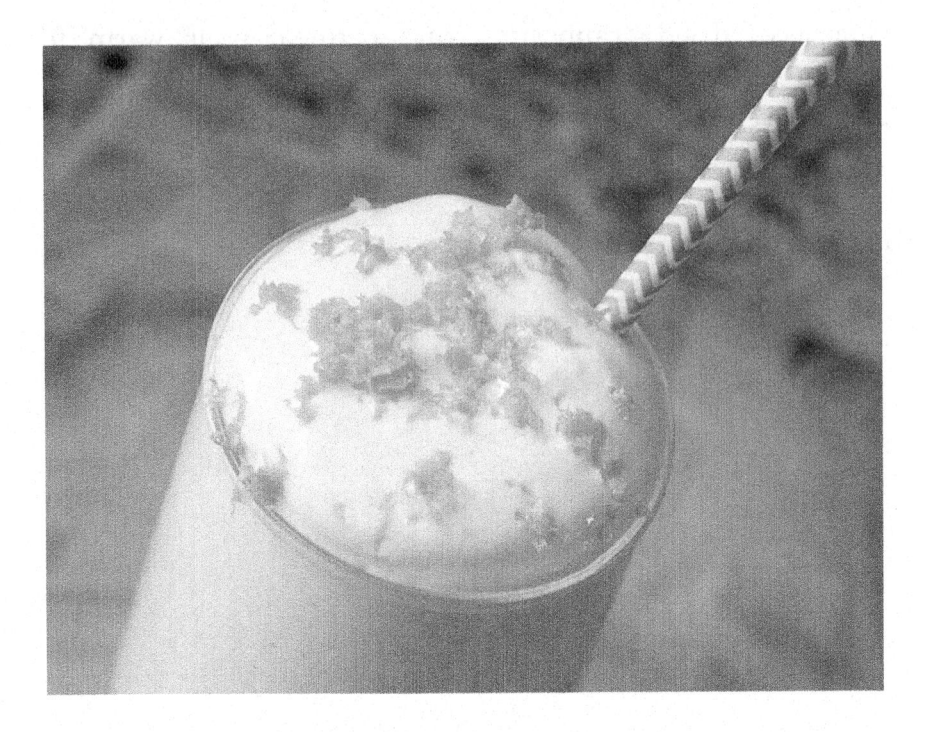

Ingredients:

- 1/2 small ripe banana
- 1 small navel orange, peeled, cut in half, pith removed
- 160ml unsweetened almond milk
- 1/4 tsp ground cinnamon
- 1 scoop vanilla protein powder
- 75g frozen mango chunks
- 2 ice cubes

Instructions:

1. Place all the ingredients in the blender.
2. Pulse until creamy and smooth.
3. The end result has to be a rich color exotic cocktail.

Prep Time: 5 min

Serves: 2

Mango Basil Smoothie

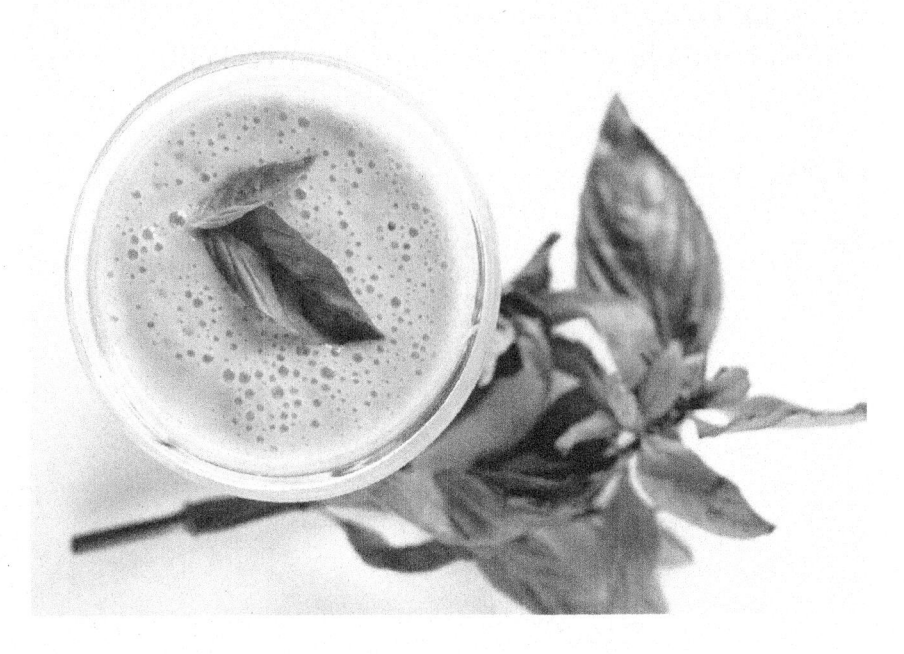

Ingredients:

- 1 mango
- 1/4 cup of basil
- 1/4 cup of spinach
- 1/2 of lime
- 1,5 of orange

Instructions:

1. Squeeze orange and lime juice, peel and cut a mango.
2. Place all the ingredients in the blender. Pulse until creamy and smooth.
3. The end result has to be a rich green color exotic cocktail.

Prep Time: 5 min

Serves: 1

Minty Mango Smoothie

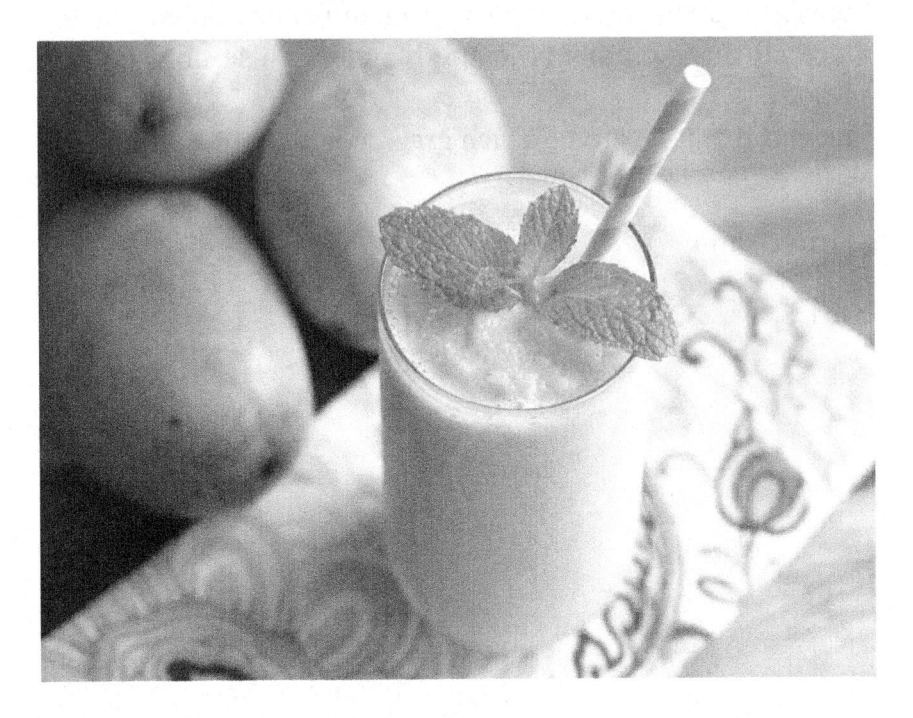

Ingredients:

- 1 mango
- fresh juice of half of the orange
- Handful of fresh mint leaves
- half of banana
- 50g ginger syrup
- 3 cubes of ice

Instructions:

1. If you can, find frozen pieces of mango, if not just place peeled and cut mango in the fridge for half an hour before blending.
2. Mix everything together, pulse until the mint is fully grounded. Enjoy!

Prep Time: 5 min

Serves: 1-2

Blueberry, Coconut & Peanut Butter Smoothie

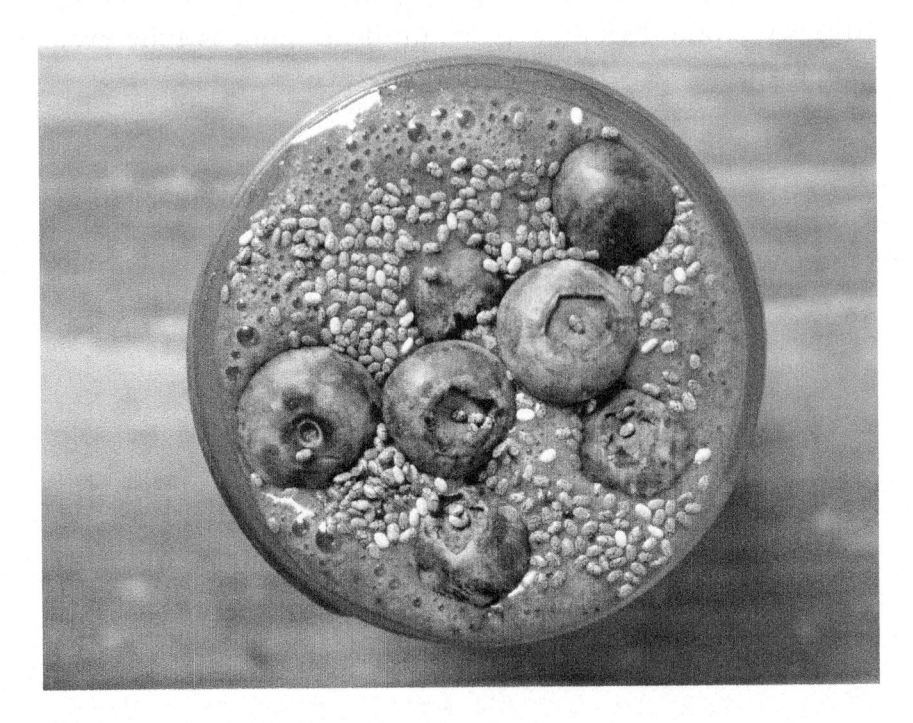

Ingredients:

- 300g frozen blueberries
- 1L coconut milk
- 2 tbsp smooth peanut butter
- 4 tbsp chia seeds
- 4 tbsp linseeds
- 1 tsp maca powder

Instructions:

1. Place everything in the blender and pulse until finely ground. The end result has to be smooth.
2. Enjoy!

Prep Time: 5 min

Serves: 2

Almond Smoothie Berry

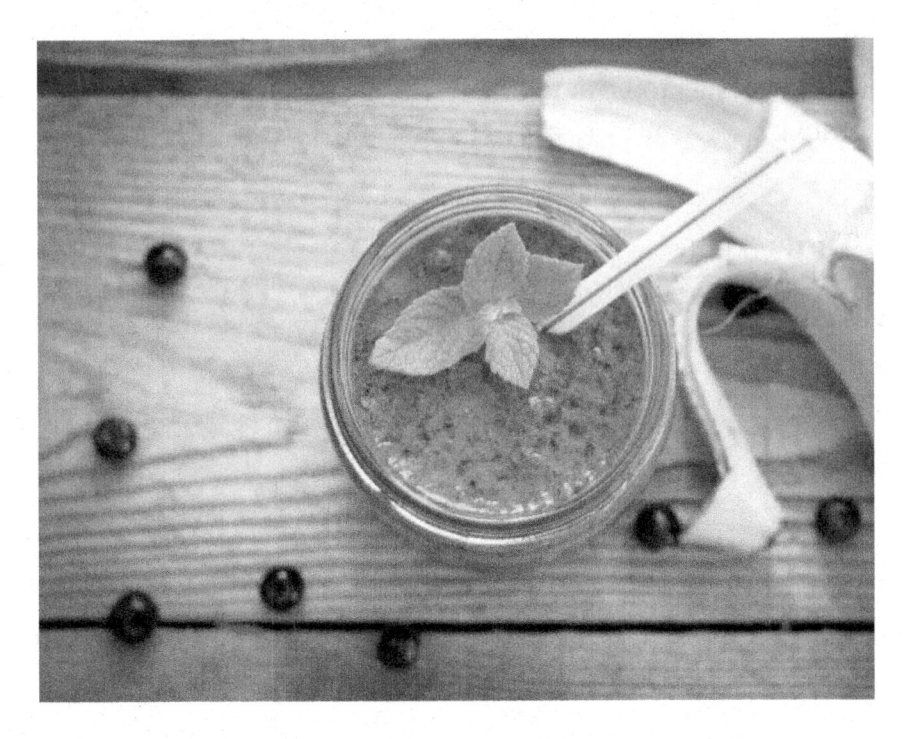

Ingredients:

- 1/2 small ripe banana, peeled, cut in half
- 250ml almond milk
- 1 tbsp almond butter
- 125g frozen mixed berries

Instructions:

Place all ingredients into and place them in the blender in the order listed.

Prep Time: 5 min

Serves: 2

Protein Smoothie

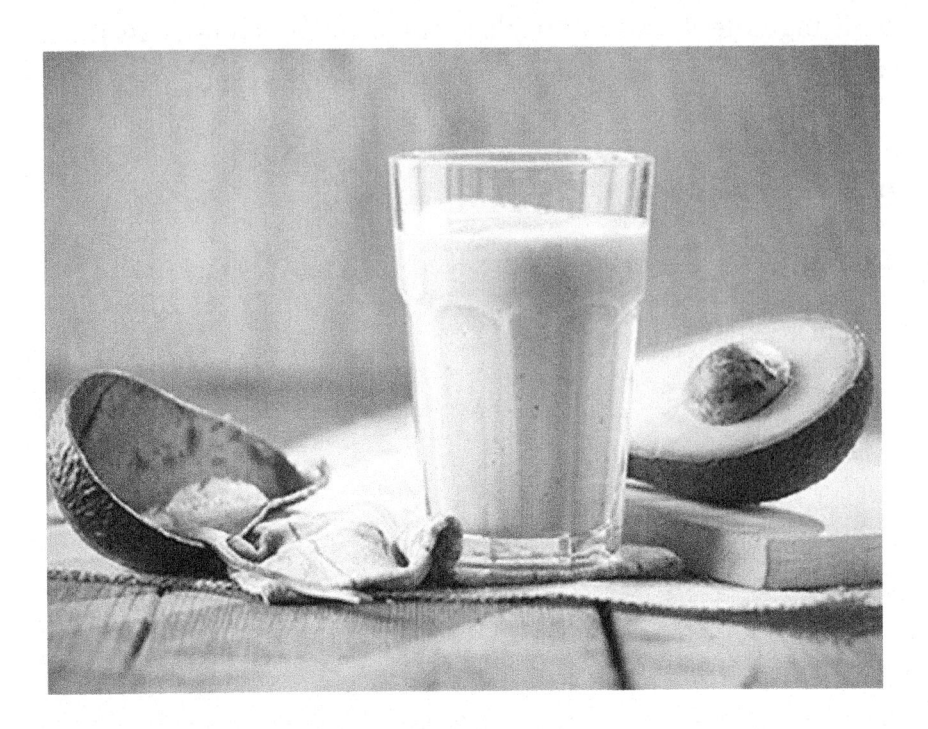

Ingredients:

- 600ml almond milk
- 2 tbsp chia seeds
- 2 tbsp hemp protein
- 1 tbsp peanut butter
- 1 banana, frozen
- 1/4 avocado
- 1 tbsp gluten-free oats
- One handful of frozen spinach

Instructions:

1. Place all of the ingredients in the large blender cup.
2. Blend until smooth.
3. Serve and enjoy.

Prep Time: 7 min

Serves: 2

Smoothie Bowls

Several smoothie recipes that would change your breakfast forever.

Rich and tasty smoothie cups are a great choice for breakfast. This is the same smoothie, but poured into a bowl and decorated with nutritious fillings. Here you will find ??? Smoothie recipes that take no more than 10 minutes of your time.

Protein Power Smoothie Bowl

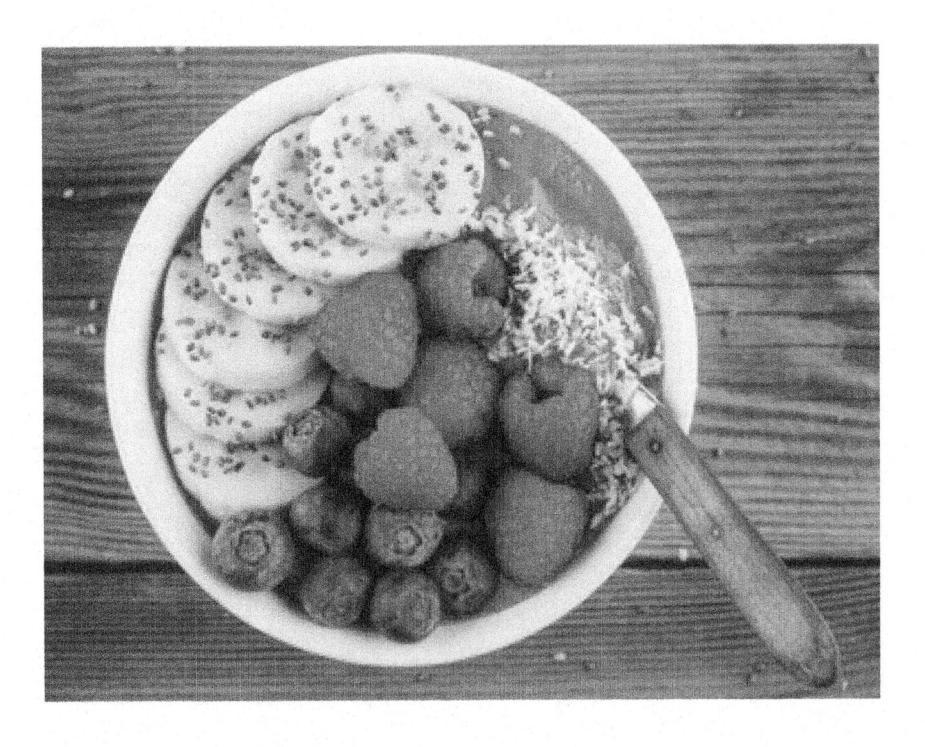

Ingredients:

- ½ cup of coconut water
- ½ cup (frozen or fresh) pineapple
- ¼ cup frozen peas
- 1 cucumber, chopped
- 1 teaspoon spirulina
- 1/2 tsp vanilla extract
- 1 handful mint
- Optional: 1/2 scoop protein powder, 1 teaspoon honey or teaspoon stevia (for sweetness)
- **Toppings:** shredded coconut, chia seeds, hemp seeds, strawberries, blueberries, raspberries, banana

Instructions:

1. Place all the ingredients into a high-speed blender and blend well.
2. Add smoothie mixture to a bowl and top with your desired toppings.

Prep Time: 10 minutes

Serves: 1

Acai Breakfast Bowl

Acai has a naturally tart flavor which goes well with other fruits and nuts.

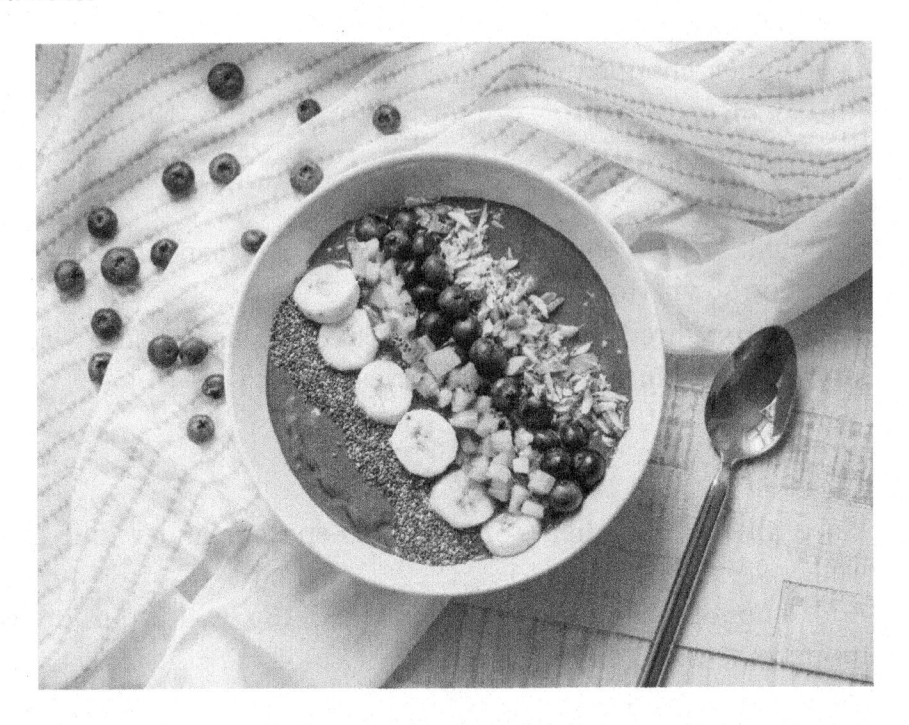

Ingredients:

- 2 packets frozen Acai berry or 2 Tbsp of acai powder
- ½ frozen or fresh banana
- 1 cup any of frozen or fresh berries
- 1 Tbsp of cashews
- ½ cup of water
- 1 tsp of honey (optional)
- **Toppings:** Chopped brazil nuts, shredded coconut, hemp seeds, sliced kiwi fruit, chia seeds

Instructions:

1. Place all the ingredients of the acai berry mixture into a high-speed blender and blend well.
2. Place acai berry mixture into a bowl and top with your desired toppings.

Prep Time: 10 minutes

Servings: 1

Berry Yogurt Smoothie Bowl

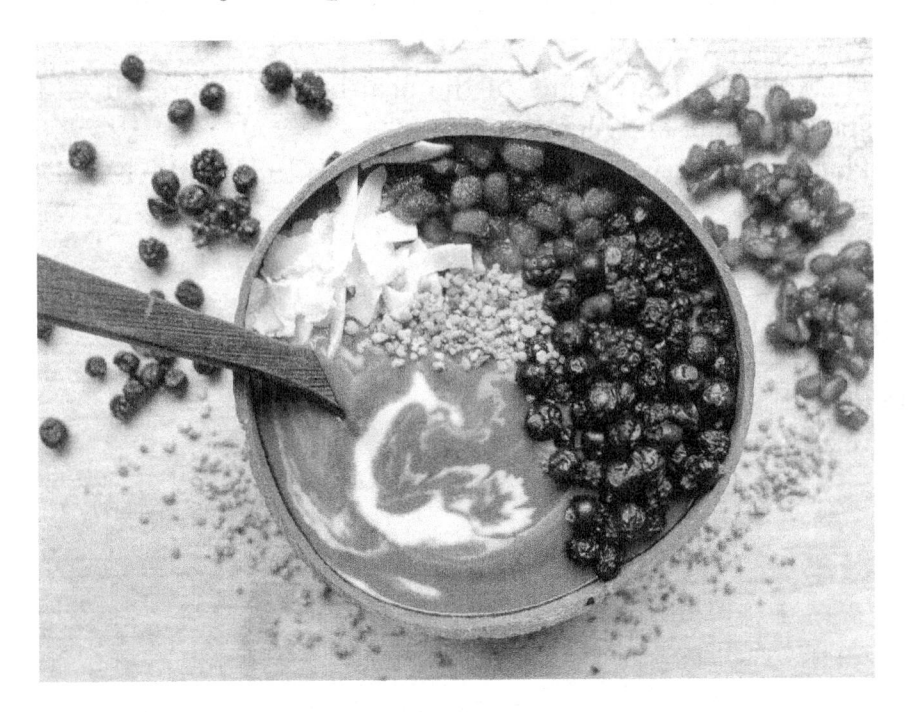

Ingredients:

- 1 frozen banana
- 75g frozen mixed berries
- 100ml apple or orange juice
- 1 tsp acai powder (optional)
- 2 tbsp yogurt (can be dairy-free)

To Decorate
- Freeze-dried berries
- Pomegranate seeds
- Bee pollen
- Coconut chips

Instructions:

1. Place the frozen banana, berries, fruit juice, and acai powder into your Ninja Kitchen blender and whizz up for about 1 minute until quite thick and smooth.
2. Pour into a bowl and swirl in the yogurt.
3. Add toppings and enjoy

Prep Time: 10 minutes

Servings: 1

Chocolate Almond Smoothie Bowl

You can add protein powder bump up the protein content on this breakfast bowl.

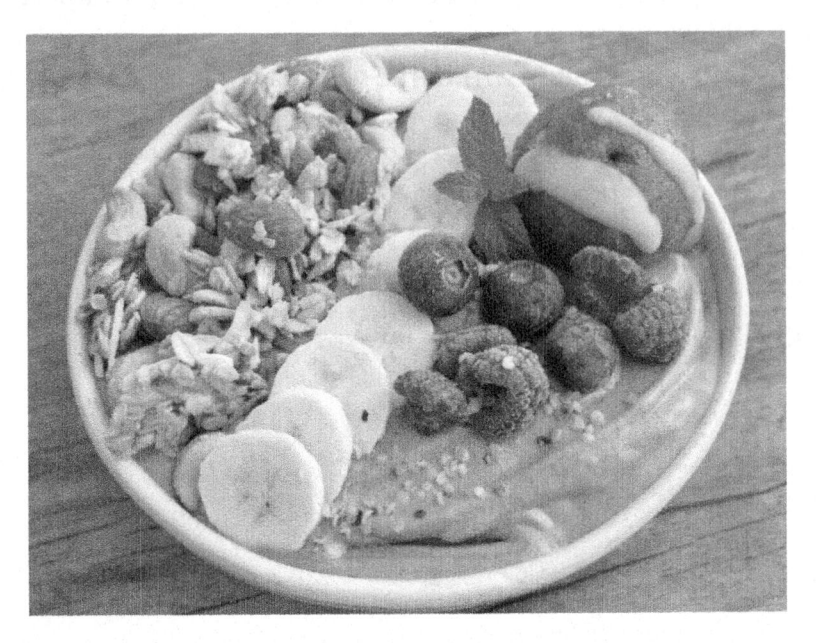

Ingredients:

- 1 banana frozen
- ½ cup of blueberries
- 1 handful of spinach
- 2 Tbsp almond butter
- 1 Tbsp cacao powder
- 1/2 tsp vanilla extract
- ½ cup of almond milk
- Stevia to taste or 1 date
- Optional: 1 scoop protein powder
- **Toppings**: chopped nuts, shredded coconut, chia seeds, cacao nibs, blueberries or strawberries

Instructions:

1. Place all the ingredients into a high-speed blender and blend well.
2. Place chocolate mixture into a bowl and top with your desired toppings.

Prep Time: 10 minutes

Servings: 1

Chocolate smoothie bowl with coconut

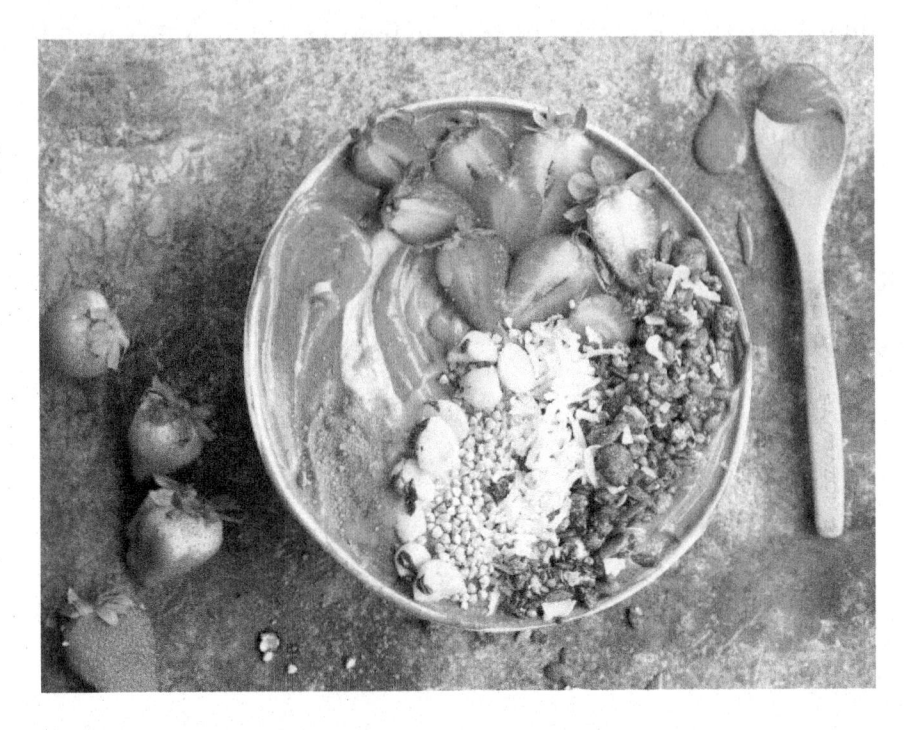

Ingredients:

- 2 cut, frozen bananas
- 1 tablespoon of almond butter
- 1—2 tablespoons of cocoa
- 1 cup of coconut milk
- 1 cup of rice or almond milk
- ***Toppings:*** 3 strawberries, 1 tablespoon of coconut chips, a handful of macadamia nuts, 1/2 teaspoon of poppy seeds

Instructions:

Place all the ingredients in the blender, pulse until creamy and smooth. Pour in the deep bowl and decorate with the toppings as desired

Prep Time: 5 minutes

Servings: 1

Berry Smoothie Bowl

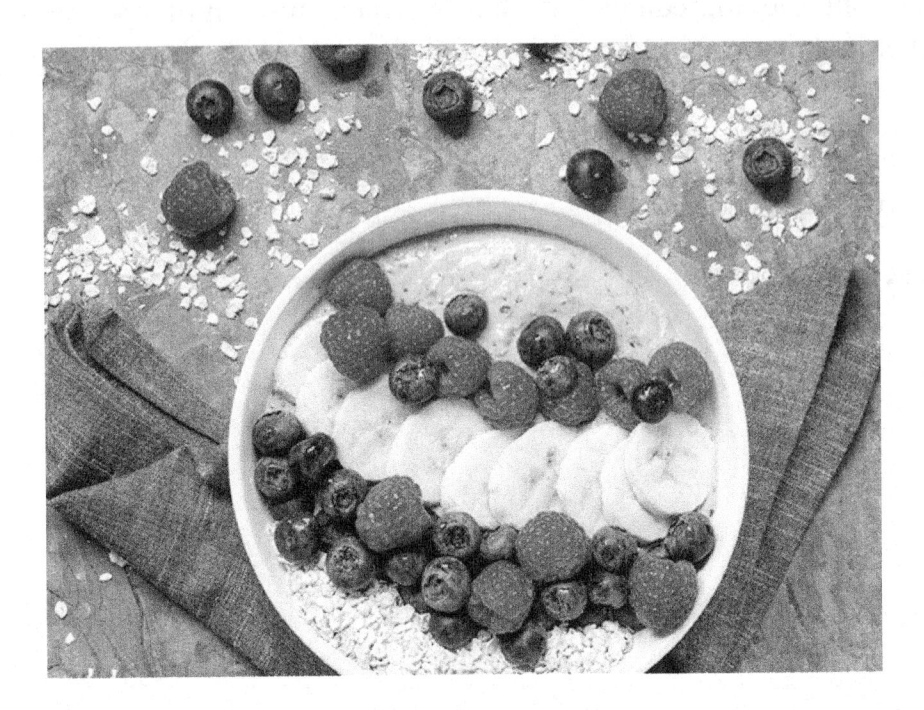

Ingredients:

- 1 banana
- 1/2 avocado
- 1 cup of frozen raspberries and blueberries
- 1/4 cup of almond milk
- 1 tablespoon of grounded flax seeds
- ***Toppings:*** banana, berries, almonds

Instructions:

Mix all the ingredient in the blender, until creamy. Pour in the bowl and add toppings. Enjoy!

Prep Time: 7 min

Serves: 1

Green Smoothie Bowl

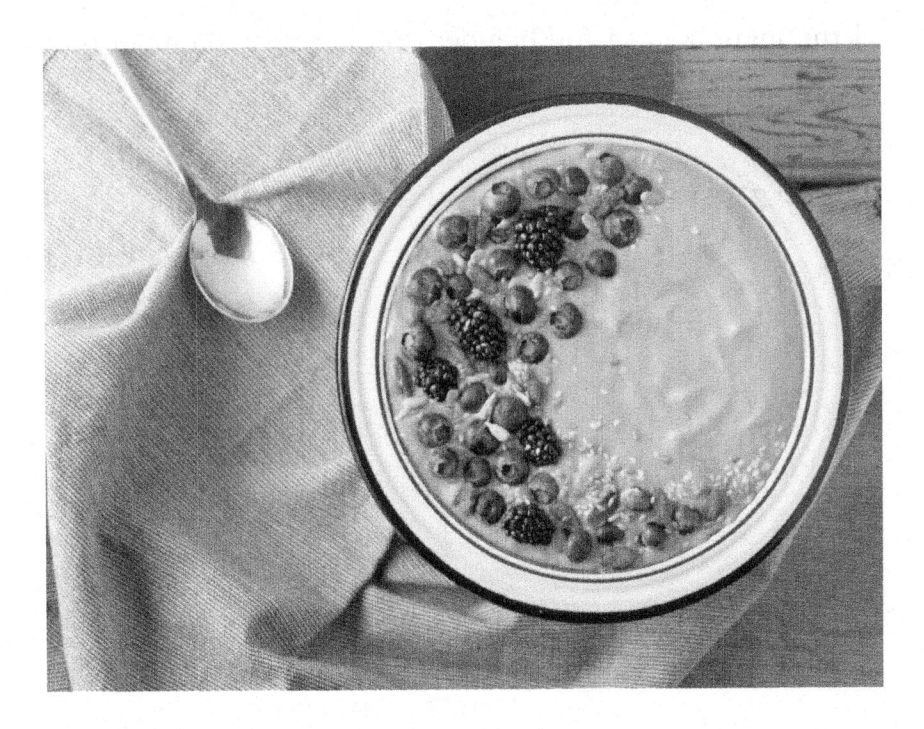

Ingredients:

- 1/2 avocado
- 2 middle bananas
- 1 cup of frozen raspberry
- 2 handful of spinach
- 1 handful of kale or parsley
- 1 1/2 or 2 cups of almond milk or coconut water
- Toppings: any berries, goji berries, sunflower seeds, flax seeds, sesame seeds

Instructions:

1. Place all the ingredients in the blender and pulse until creamy and smooth. Distribute the smoothie evenly in the serving bowls. and decorate with toppings.
2. Eat with the spoon and enjoy!

Prep Time: 10 min

Servings: 2

Green Smoothie Bowl with Peanut butter

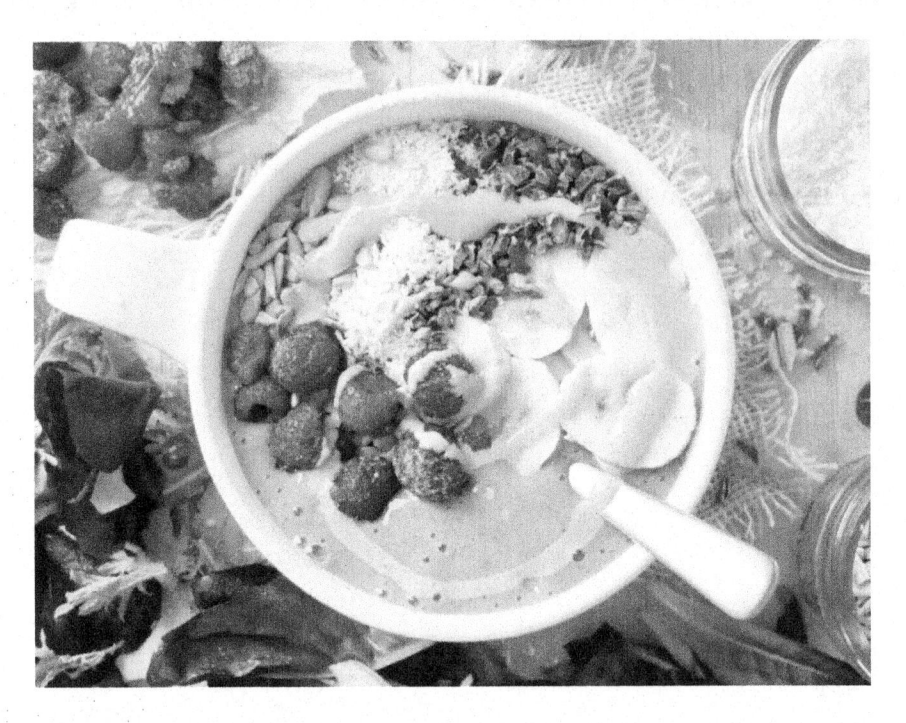

Ingredients:

- 2 bananas
- a cup of frozen fruits(pineapple or peach)
- tablespoons of flax seeds
- tablespoons of peanut butter
- cup of spinach
- 1/2—1 cup of vegetable milk

Toppings:

- 1 banana
- 1/2 cup of raspberries or other berries
- 2 tablespoons of sunflower seeds
- 2 tablespoons of coconut chips
- 2 tablespoons of ground cocoa beans
- 1 tablespoon of peanut butter

Instructions:

1. Mix all the ingredients together until fully blended. Pour in the bowl and decorate as you like.
2. Enjoy!

Prep Time: 10 min

Servings: 2

Blue Smoothie Bowl

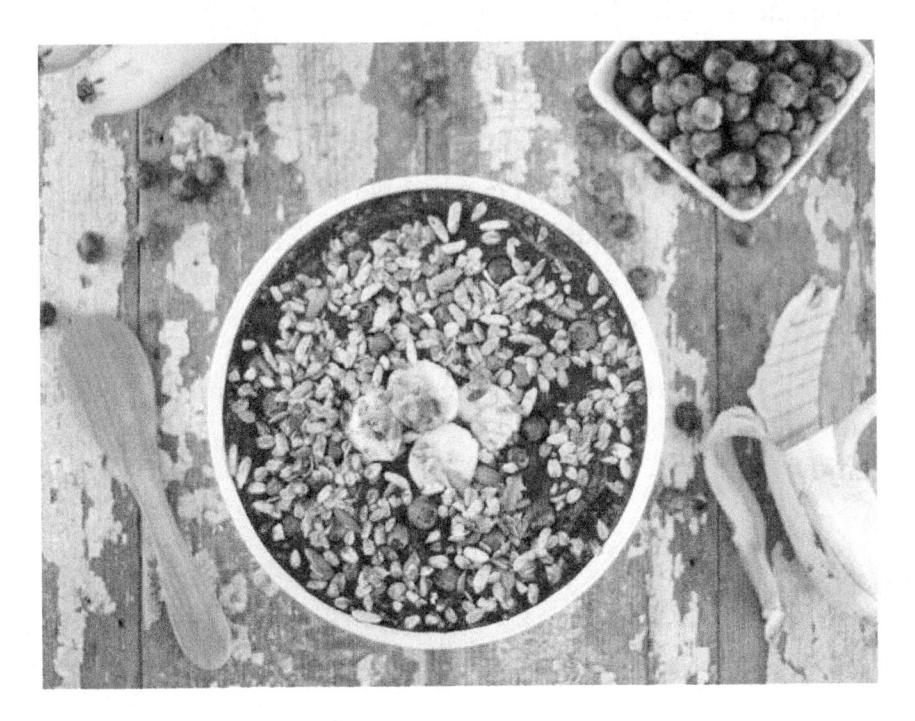

Ingredients:

- 3 cups of spinach
- frozen banana
- a bowl of frozen blueberries
- 1/2 cup of almond milk or water
- 1/2 cup of ice
- 1 tablespoon of almond butter
- pinch of cinnamon
- stevia or other sweeteners
- 1 teaspoon of poppy seeds
- Toppings: your favorite granola

Instructions:

1. Place everything in a blender and process to obtain a smooth liquid.
2. Pour in the bowl and sprinkle with granola.

Prep Time: 10 min

Servings: 1

Diner

When it comes to turning a full-fledged dish into a smoothie, it is important that there are vegetables in the smoothie, some fruit for sweetness and taste, healthy fats and proteins; basically, everything you find in food. This helps to ensure not only satiety but also that it is well balanced.

Healthy Brain smoothies

This smoothie is made up of brain-friendly but tasty ingredients that help maintain healthy blood vessels. You can add vegetable protein for added balance and nutrients.

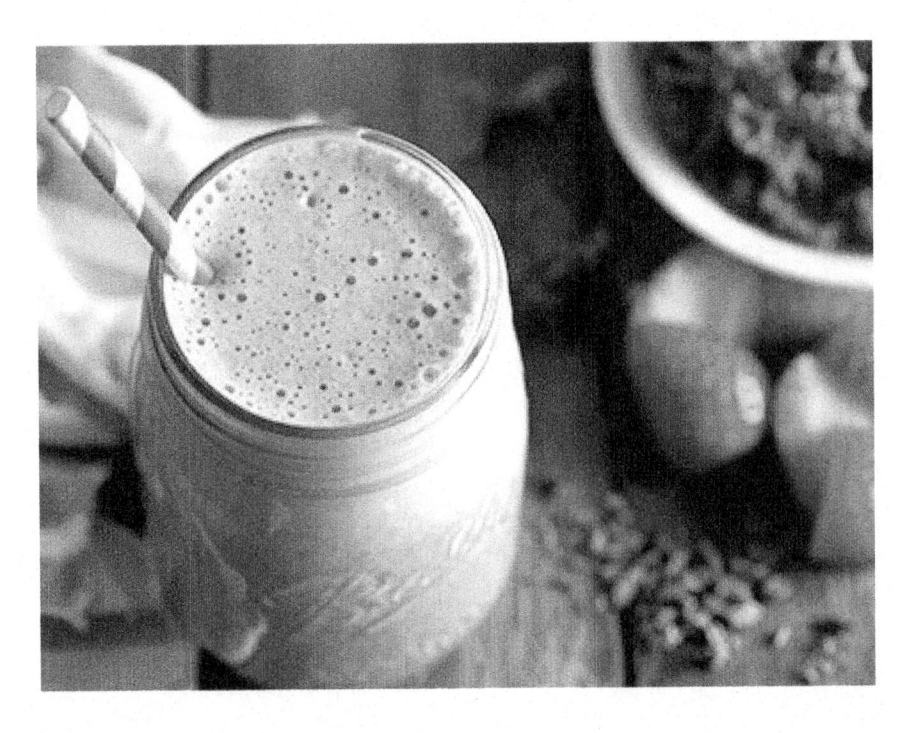

Ingredients:

- 5 strawberries, tops removed
- 2 handfuls of cabbage
- 2 tablespoons of cocoa beans (preferably raw)
- Dash each: turmeric and cinnamon
- 8 oz hemp milk
- (optional) 1 scoop of vegetable protein

Instructions:

1. Wash and cook the ingredients.
2. Add ingredients to the blender and mix for 45-60 seconds or until mixed.
3. Serve and enjoy!

Prep Time: 5-10 minutes

Servings: 1

Berry Protein Shake

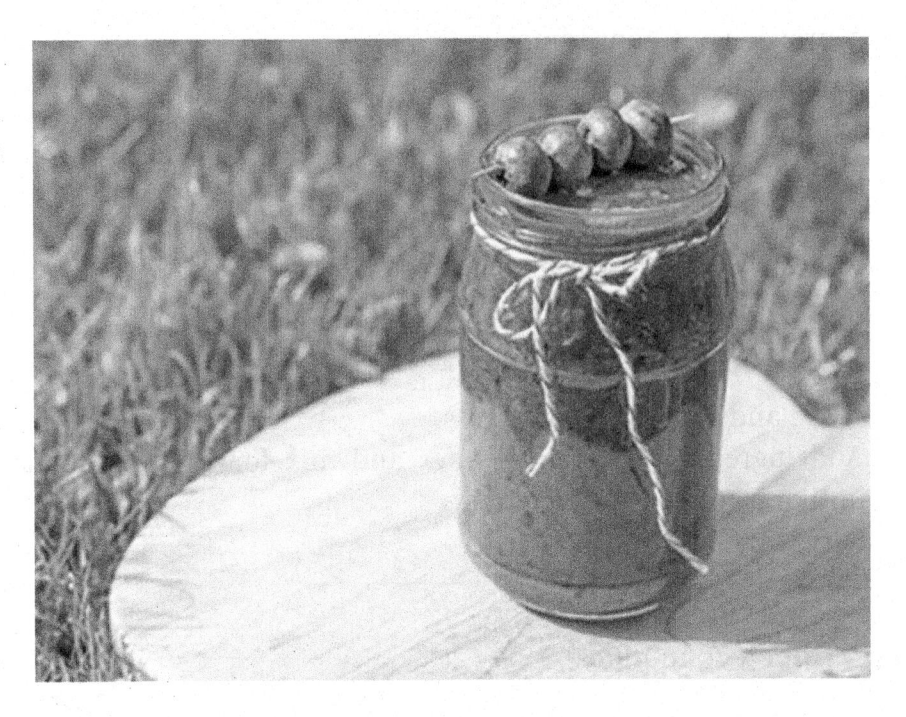

Ingredients:

- cup (250 ml) almond milk
- scoop plant-based protein powder or 3 tbsp hemp seeds
- 1/2 cup (50 g) frozen blueberries
- 1/3 avocado
- kale leaves
- 1/2 tsp vanilla extract

Instructions:

1. Wash the kale leaves well.
2. Add ingredients to a blender and blend on high for 45-60 seconds until smooth.

Prep Time: 5 minutes

Servings: 1

Protein Smoothie

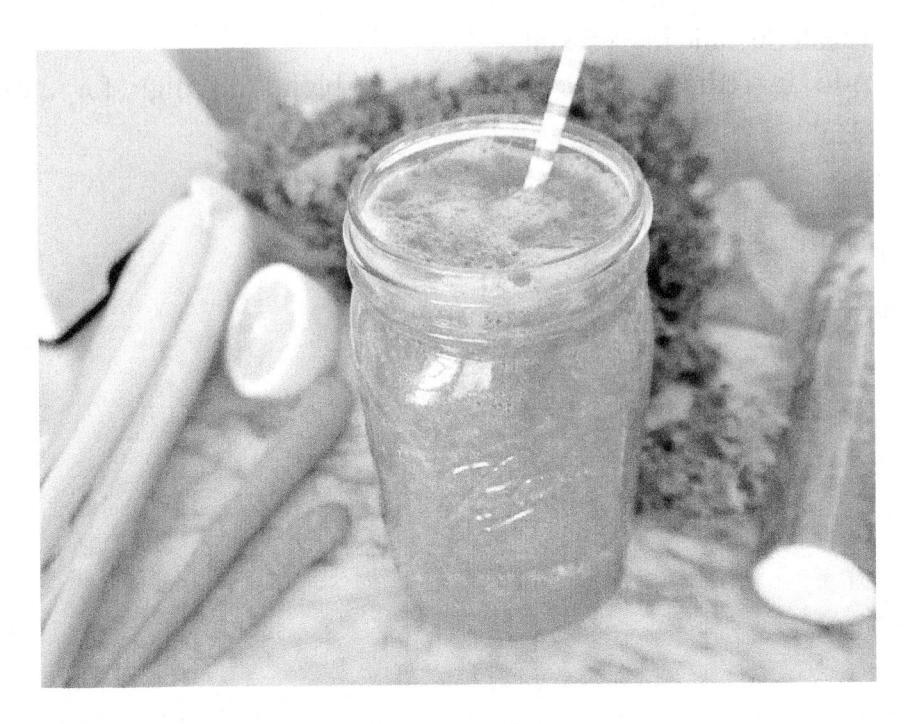

Ingredients:

- ½ banana
- carrot
- 1 stalk celery
- 1 cup (30 g) spinach
- 1 inch (2.5 cm) piece of ginger
- ¼ lemon, peeled
- 1 tsp coconut oil
- 1 scoop plant-based protein
- 1 cup (250 ml) water or unsweetened almond milk

Instructions:

1. Wash and prepare ingredients.
2. Add all ingredients to the blender and blend on high for 45-60 seconds or until well mixed.
3. Serve and enjoy!

Prep Time: 5 min

Servings: 1

Simple Protein Smoothie

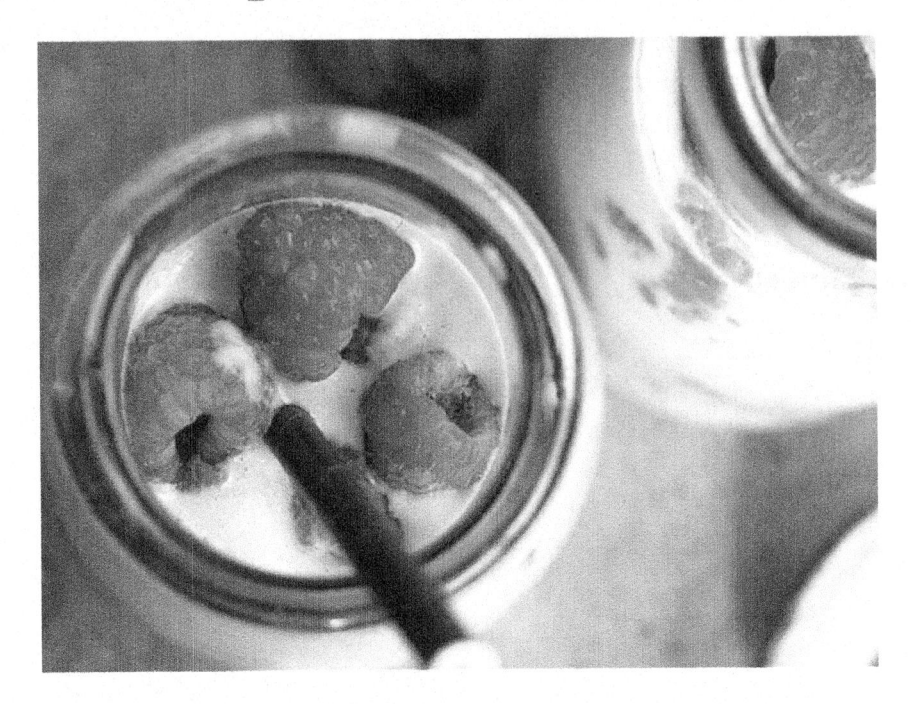

Ingredients:

- ¾ cup (90 g) raspberries
- cup (30 g) spinach
- 1 scoop plant-based protein, or sprouted rice or hemp protein
- 1 cup (250 ml) unsweetened almond or coconut milk
- 1/3 avocado or 1-2 tablespoons of almond or cashew butter.
- 5 ice cubes

Instructions:

1. Wash all produce well.
2. Add ingredients to a blender and blend on high for 45 – 60 seconds until smooth.

Prep Time: 7 min

Servings: 1

Simple green smoothie

Hemp seeds will make the smoothie a more balanced and complete source of vegetable protein, and will also contribute to satiety.

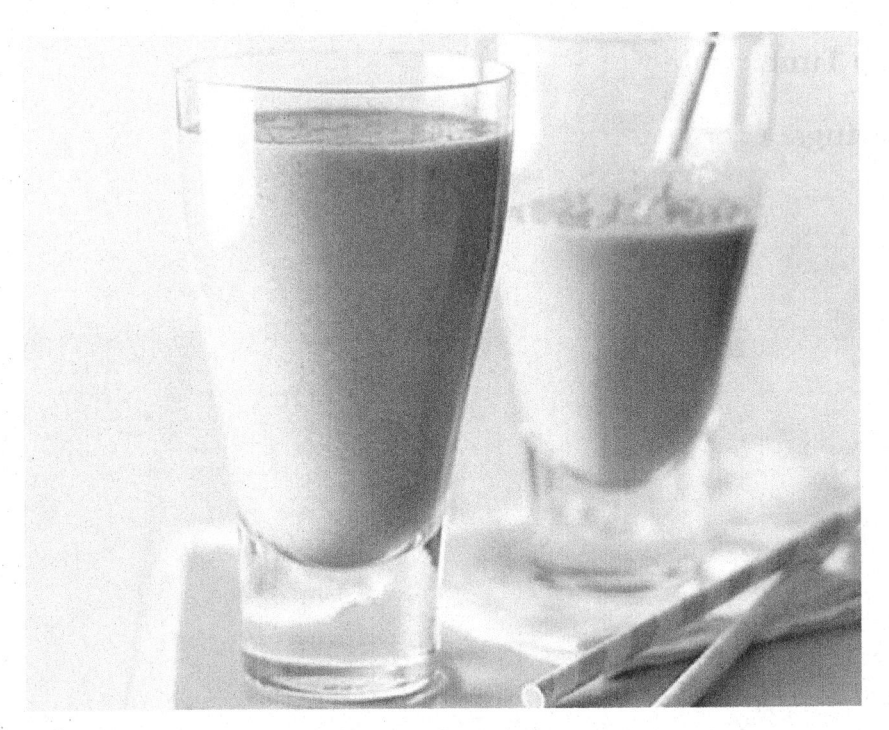

Ingredients:

- cup (250 ml) of almond milk, unsweetened
- pear, pith
- cabbage leaves
- tablespoons of hemp seeds
- 1 teaspoon honey (optional)

Instructions:

1. Wash and cook the ingredients.
2. Add ingredients to the blender and mix well for 45-60 seconds.
3. Serve and enjoy!

Prep Time: 5 min

Servings: 1

Full Protein Smoothie

Instead of pea protein, you can use another type of vegetable protein, such as brown rice protein, hemp heart, or others!

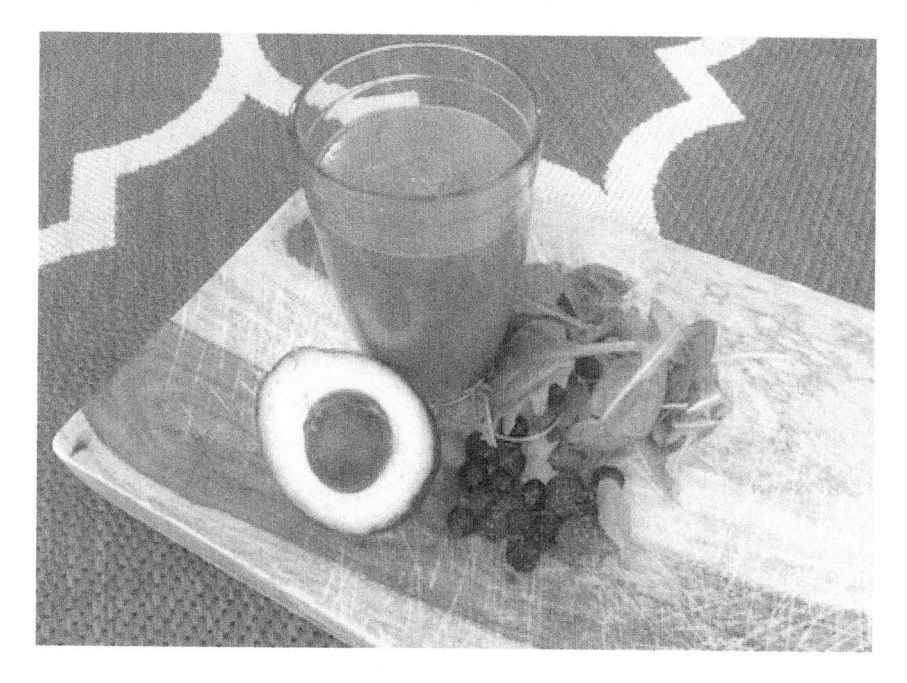

Ingredients:

- ½ avocado
- teaspoon almond oil
- 1 spoon (portion) of pea protein
- ½ banana
- ½ cup berries
- 1 handful (cup) of arugula or any greens

Instructions:

1. Wash and cook the ingredients.
2. Add the ingredients to the blender and stir over medium heat for 30-60 seconds or until mixed.
3. Serve and enjoy!

Prep Time: 5 min

Servings: 1

Low-Sugar Smoothie

In this cocktail a lot of fiber and healthy fats, but minimally carbohydrates.

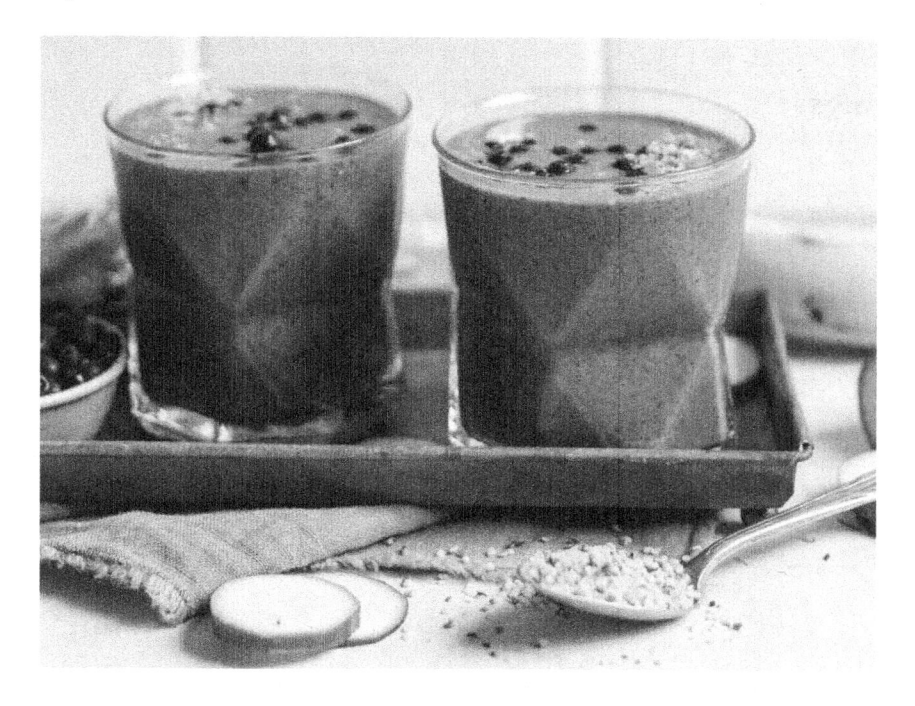

Ingredients:

- ½ cup of coconut water
- 1 cup sliced and frozen zucchini
- ½ avocado
- ½ cup frozen blueberries
- 1 tablespoon almond oil
- 1 teaspoon hemp seed
- pinch of sea salt

Instructions:

Place all ingredients in a blender and blend until smooth. Enjoy!

Prep Time: 10 min

Servings: 1

Cauliflower Smoothie

Looking for all the benefits of a green smoothie without the green and without the added sugars from banana. Try a cauliflower smoothie offering a creamy and thick texture.

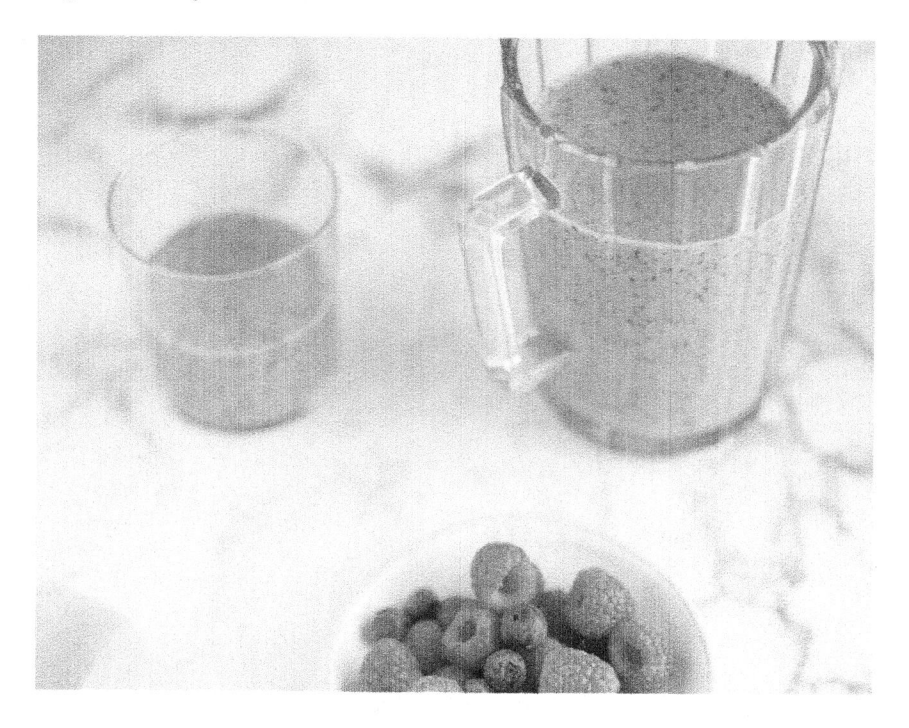

Ingredients:

- Tbsp almond butter
- 10 oz coconut water
- 1/4 cup frozen blueberries
- 1/4 cup frozen raspberries
- 1/2 cup frozen cauliflower (any cut)*
- 1 scoop (serving) plant-based protein (optional)

Instructions:

1. Combine all ingredients in a blender
2. Blend on high until well mixed for about 45-60 seconds
3. Serve and enjoy

Prep Time: 5-10 min

Servings: 1

Green Coconut Smoothie

This smoothie is well balanced due to the healthy fat. and a little protein too.

To make this smoothie a complete meal, add your favorite plant-based protein to round it out!

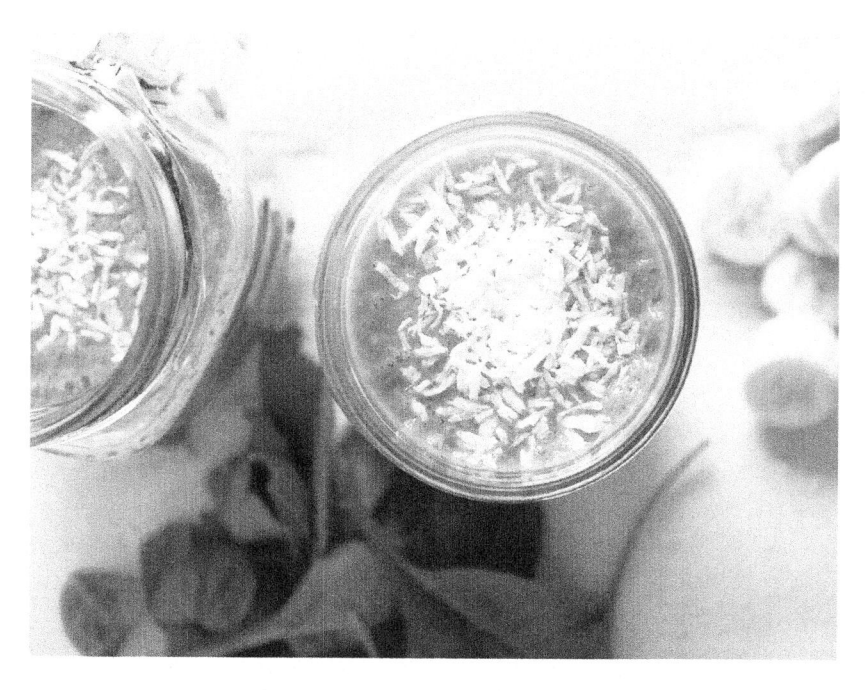

Ingredients:

- banana
- 1/3 avocado
- Tbsp coconut flakes
- Tbsp spirulina or chlorella (blue-green algae)
- Dash dried turmeric
- handfuls spinach
- 8-10 oz hemp or almond milk

Instructions:

1. Wash and prepare ingredients.
2. Add ingredients through the blender and blend on high for 45-60 seconds or until smooth.
3. Serve and enjoy!

Prep Time: 5 min

Servings: 1

Banana Raspberry Smoothie

This rich smoothie is naturally sweetened from beet and banana. Beets are a good source of folic acid and contain vitamins A, C, choline, iodine, manganese, potassium, and fiber. Raspberries are high in antioxidants, vitamin C and contain potassium, niacin, and iron.

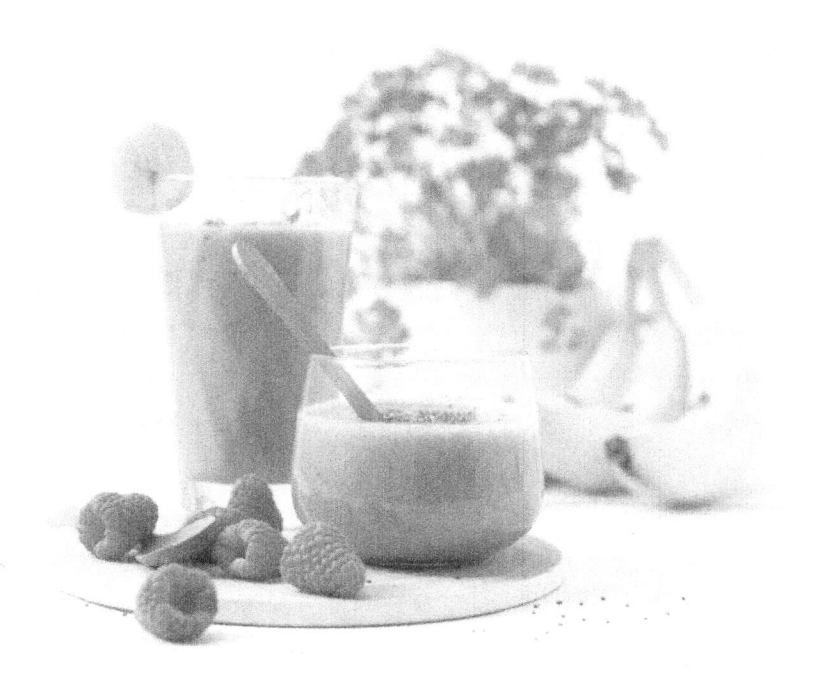

Ingredients:

- raw beet (peeled and thinly sliced)
- 1 cup raspberries (fresh or frozen)
- 1/2 banana
- 1 teaspoon vanilla extract
- 1.5 cups unsweetened almond milk (or whatever milk you like)
- a pinch of sea salt
- A few ice cubes (optional)

Instructions:

1. Wash and prepare ingredients.
2. Combine all the ingredients in a blender and blend on high for 1-2 minutes or until well mixed.
3. Enjoy!

Prep Time: 10 min

Servings: 1

Green Detox

Can a detox diet harm your body??

By drastically reducing the caloric content of food, you stress the body and deprive it of essential nutrients.

How to cleanse the body without depriving it of essential nutrients? It's easy with a perfectly made smoothie.

Leafy green vegetables are an important part of a healthy diet. They're packed with vitamins, minerals, and fiber but low in calories. Eating a diet rich in leafy greens can offer numerous health benefits including reduced risk of obesity, heart disease, high blood pressure, and mental decline

Here you are going to find easy recipes, that will include greens every day in a year.

Celery and Beet Juice

Not everyone like the taste of celery, but with beets or apple, celery becomes milder.

Ingredients:

- 1 middle beet
- 3—4 stack of celery
- 1 carrot
- 2 apples
- small piece of ginger

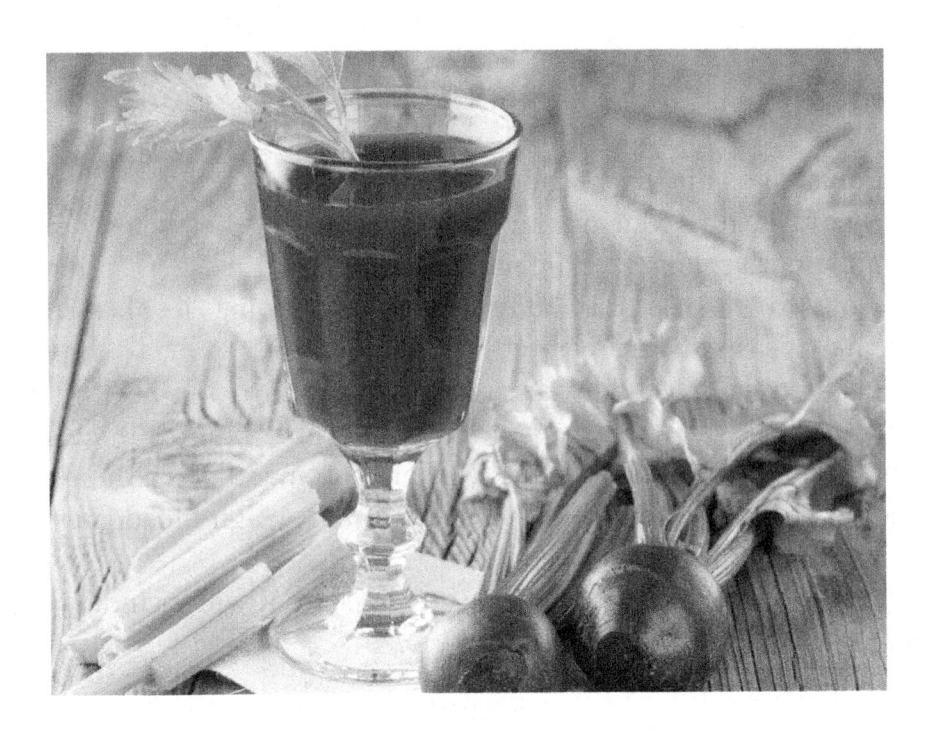

Instructions:

Place everything in the blender, and bright, nutritional smoothie is ready!!!

Prep Time: 7 min

Servings: 1-2

Green Almond Milk Smoothie

This smoothie you can drink every day!

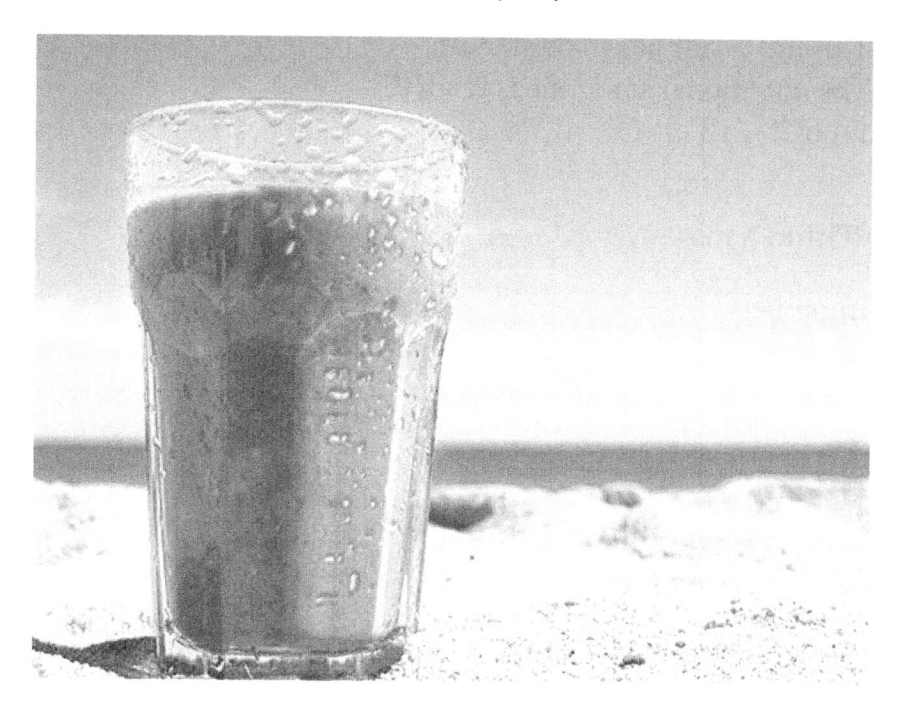

Ingredients:

- 1,5 cups of almond milk
- 1 cup of fresh spinach
- 2 frozen bananas
- 1 spoon of honey or syrup
- Lime or lemon juice

Instructions:

1. Take bananas from the freezer 5 minutes before cooking.
2. Place everything in the blender and pulse until finely ground.
3. The end result has to be smooth.
4. The nutritional smoothie is ready!!!
5. Enjoy!!

Prep Time: 5 min

Servings: 1-2

Green Citrus Juice

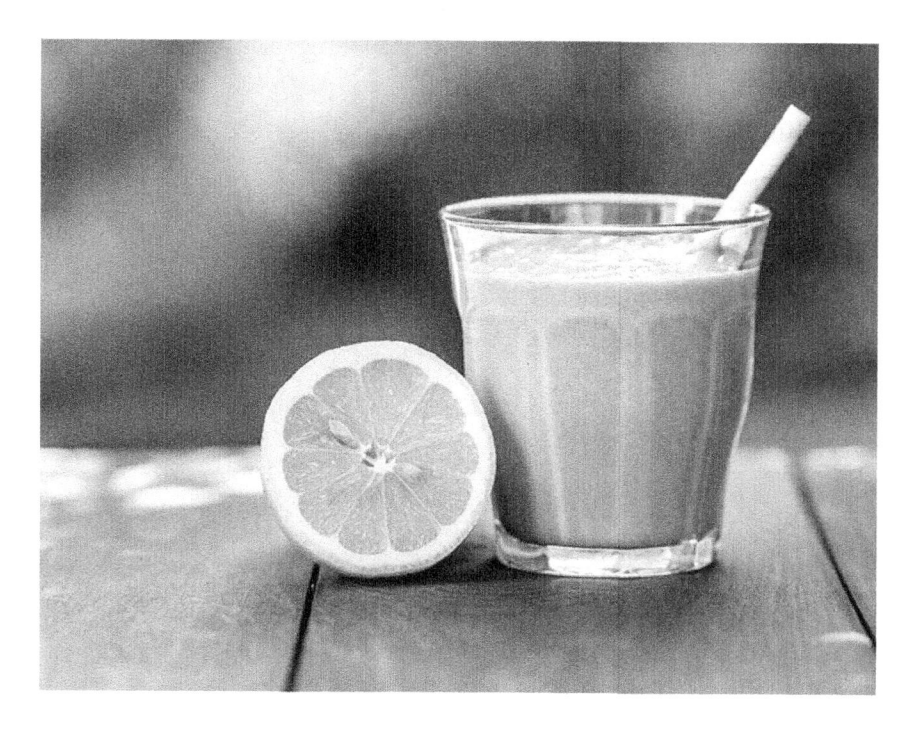

Ingredients:

- 2 mandarins
- large lime
- 1 lemon
- celery stalks
- kale leaves

Instructions:

1. Wash all produce well.
2. Peel mandarins, lemon, and lime.
3. The nutritional smoothie is ready!!!
4. Enjoy!!

Prep Time: 5 min

Servings: 1

Cold Fighting Green Smoothie

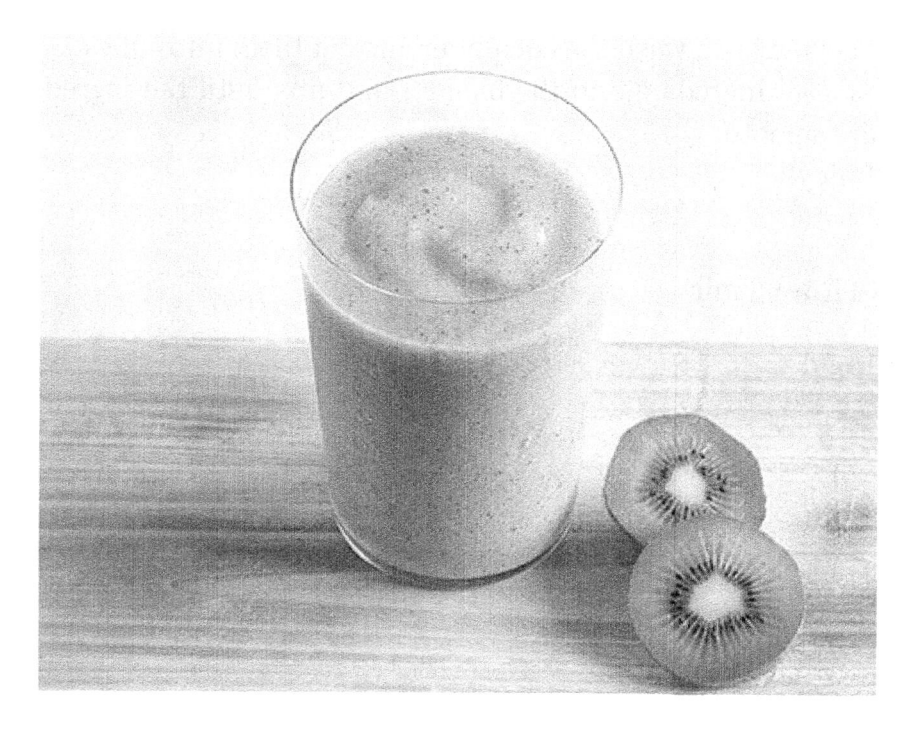

Ingredients:

- cup coconut water
- 1/4 cucumber
- tbsp live cultures natural yogurt
- 1/2 banana
- kiwis
- handfuls of spinach
- 1/4 tsp spirulina
- 10 drops Echinacea

Instructions:

1. Peel the kiwi, wash the cucumber and cut them into cubes.
2. Add all ingredients to the blender and mix until the ingredients are smooth.
3. Enjoy!!

Prep Time: 5 min

Servings: 1

Fruit and vegetable cocktail

This green smoothie contains fruits and vegetables that a powerful set of vitamins.

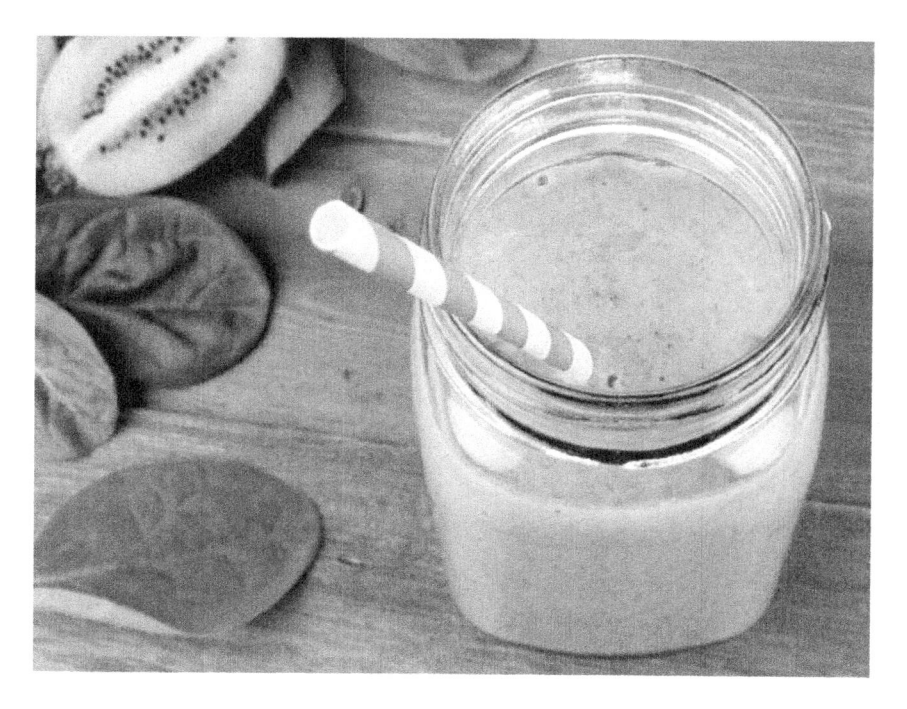

Ingredients:

- cup unsweetened almond or coconut milk (or water)
- 1 kiwi, peeled and sliced
- 1 cup pineapple, peeled and sliced (fresh or frozen)
- 1 cucumber, peeled and sliced
- 1 cup fresh spinach
- pinch of sea salt

Instructions:

Add all ingredients to a powerful blender and mix for at least until smooth.

Prep Time: 5 min

Servings: 1

Kiwi Mint Smoothie

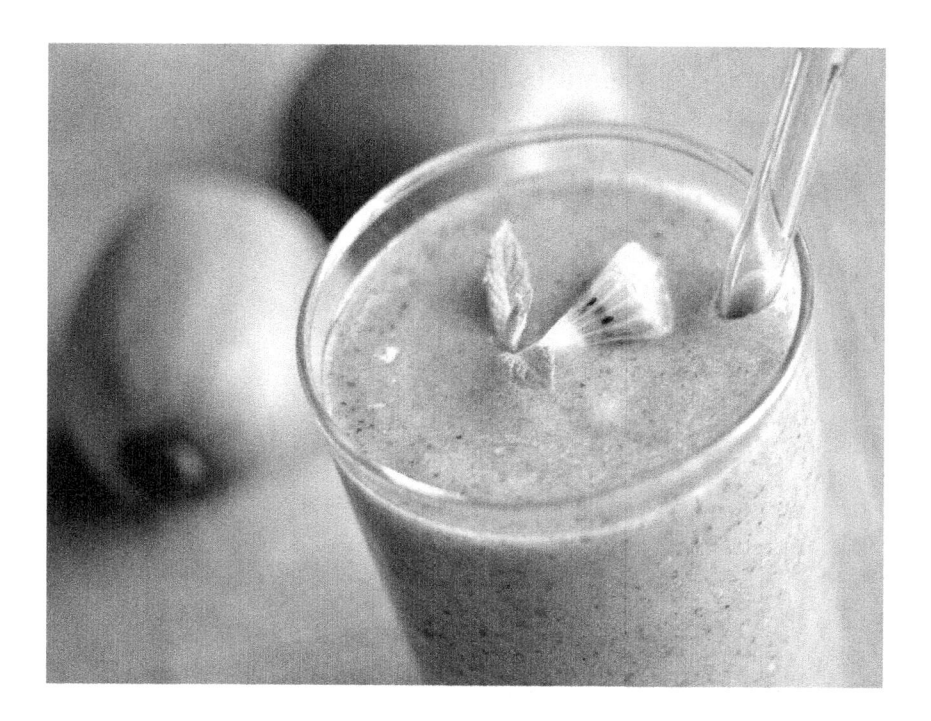

Ingredients:

- 2 kiwi
- 1/2 of green apple
- banana
- tablespoons of lemon juice
- a handful of fresh mint leaves
- cinnamon

Instructions:

1. Peel all the fruits and place them in the blender.
2. Add mint and pulse until smooth.
3. In the end, add lemon juice in order to keep the color and a pinch of cinnamon.

Prep Time: 5 min

Servings: 1

Avocado Smoothie

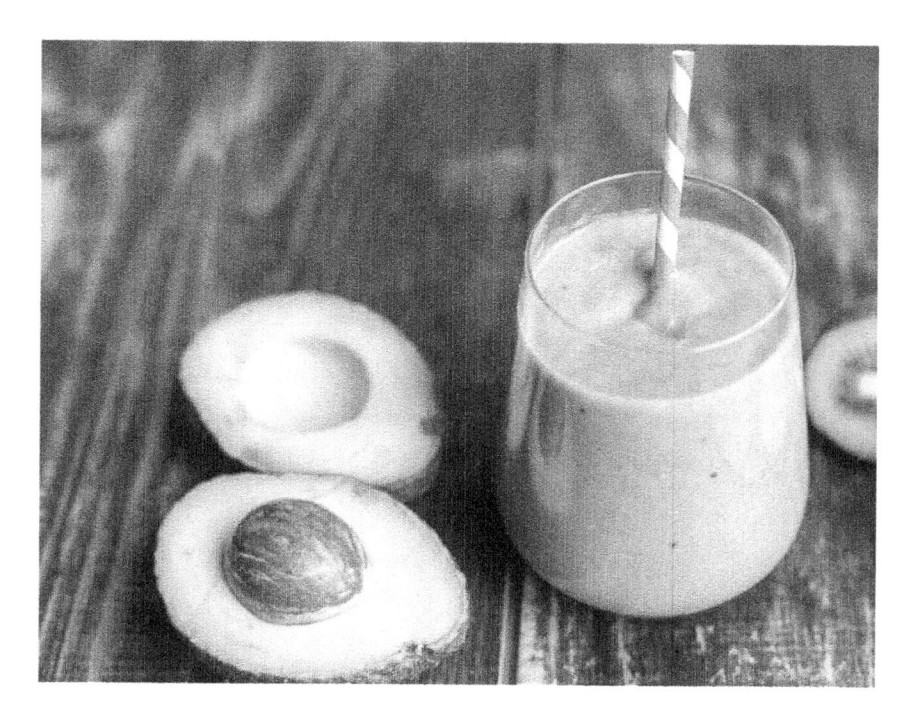

Ingredients:

- 1/2 Ripe Avocados
- 150ml Milk of your choice (I like Oat or Almond)
- 40g Coconut or Vanilla Yoghurt
- 1/2 tbsp Almond Butter
- tbsp Honey or Maple Syrup
- 1 Ice Cubes

Instructions:

1. Combine all the ingredients for the shake in a blender and blend on high for 5 minutes.
2. Pour into a cup and enjoy.

Prep Time: 5 min

Servings: 1

Green Lemonade

One of the fastest, easiest lemonades, which will be perfect for a summer day.

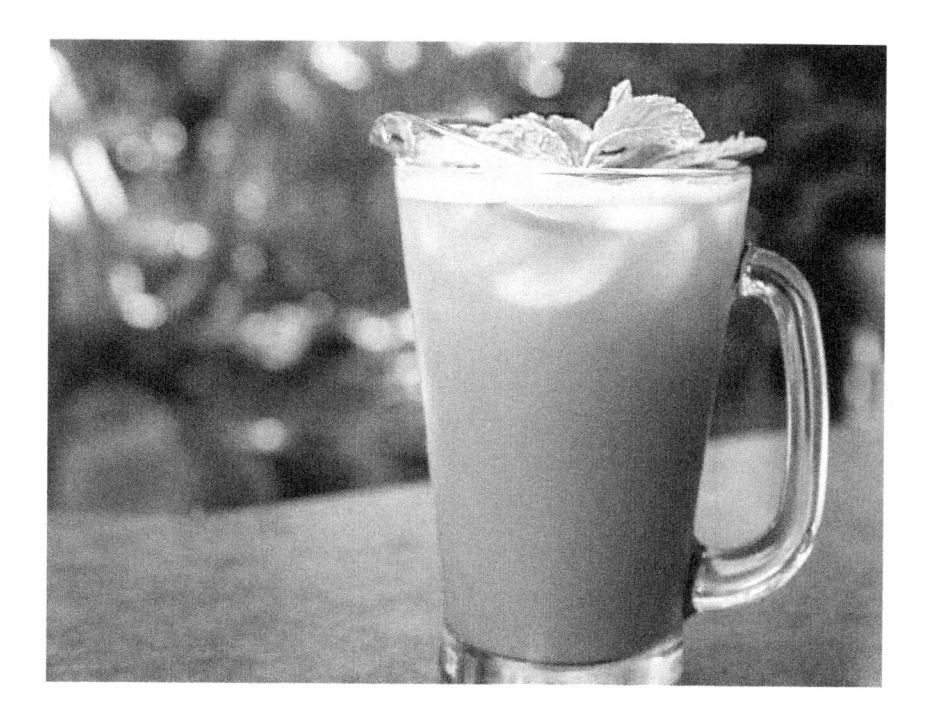

Ingredients:

- 2 cucumbers
- a handful of parsley or spinach
- ½ lemon juice
- 2 cups of water
- honey

Instructions:

Peel cucumbers and mix all the ingredient in the blender. You can place the drink in the fridge to cool.

Prep Time: 7 min

Servings: 1

Sweet Spinach Detox

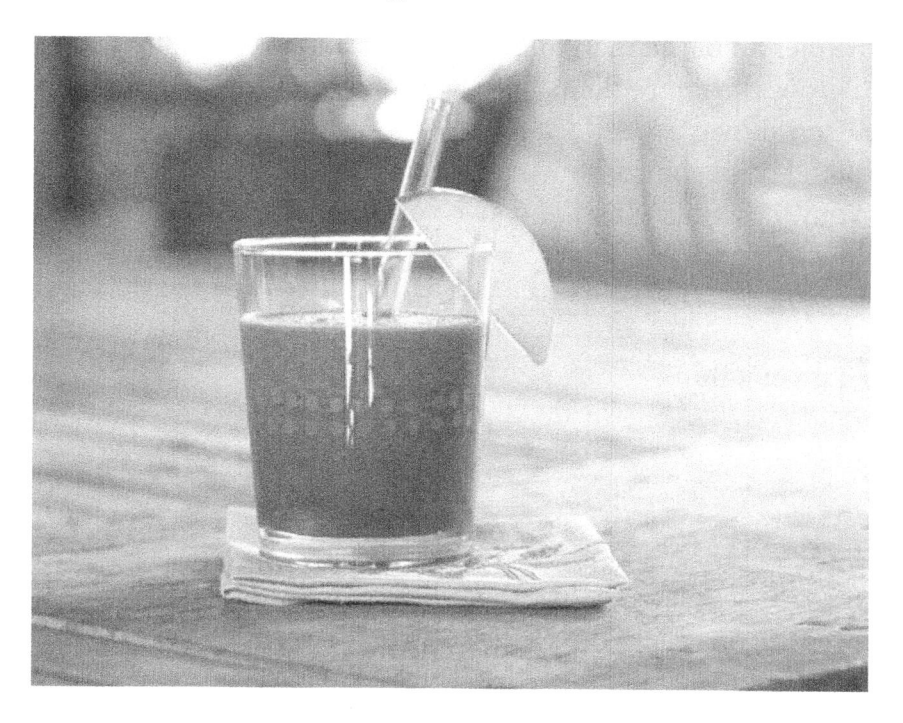

Ingredients:

- 2 apples, peeled and cored
- lemon, peeled
- 1-inch ginger, peeled
- 30g spinach
- 2tbsp agave or honey
- 100ml apple juice
- 100ml water
- 6 ice cubes

Instructions:

1. Gather all of the ingredients together and prep what you need to.
2. Throw the ingredients into your favorite blender in the order listed above.
3. Blend until your desired consistency is achieved.
4. Pour into a tall glass, and give your body a boost when it needs it most.

Prep Time: 5 min

Servings: 2

Celery Blueberry Smoothie

Best way to eat celery is to make it with a blueberry smoothie.

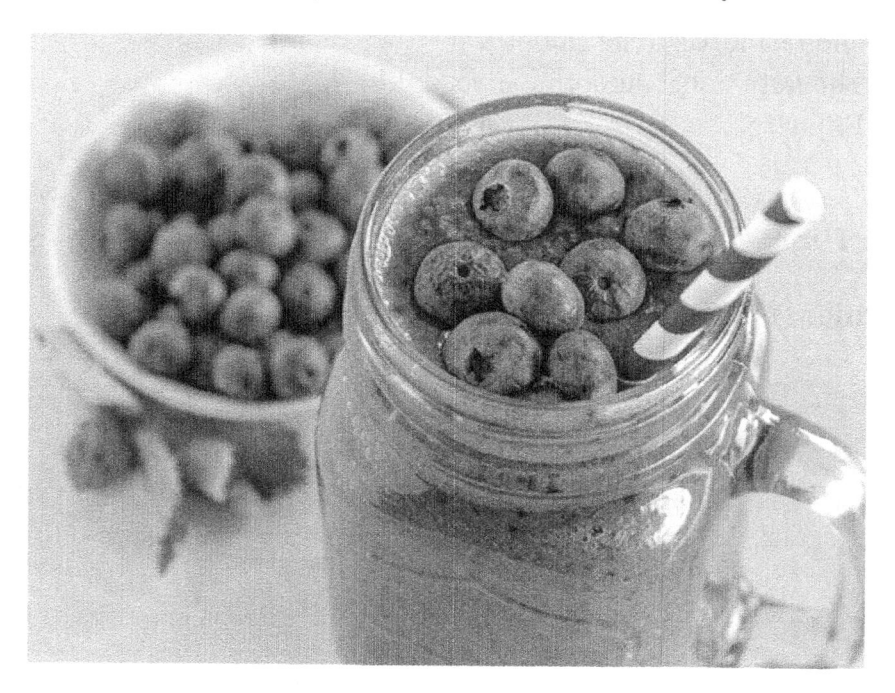

Ingredients:

- 2 bananas
- 3 tablespoons of blueberries
- ⅓ of lemon juice,
- 2—3 stack of celery
- cup of water

Instructions:

1. Wash and prepare ingredients.
2. Place everything in the blender and pulse until finely ground. The end result has to be smooth.
3. The nutritional smoothie is ready!!!
4. Enjoy!!

Prep Time: 5 min

Servings: 1-2

Warming Drinks

Smoothies are a quick and easy breakfast filled with fiber and nutrients, but when it's cold outside, you may crave something warm in the morning. Enter the warm smoothie. It's a great way to enjoy a variety of fruits and vegetables while the weather is cool. You can easily simmer ingredients on the stove and then transfer to a blender.

Spiced Apple Drink

Ginger, cardamom, and cloves help strengthen digestion, while cinnamon is known for its anti-inflammatory properties. The lemon zest and orange add extra flavor and vitamin C.

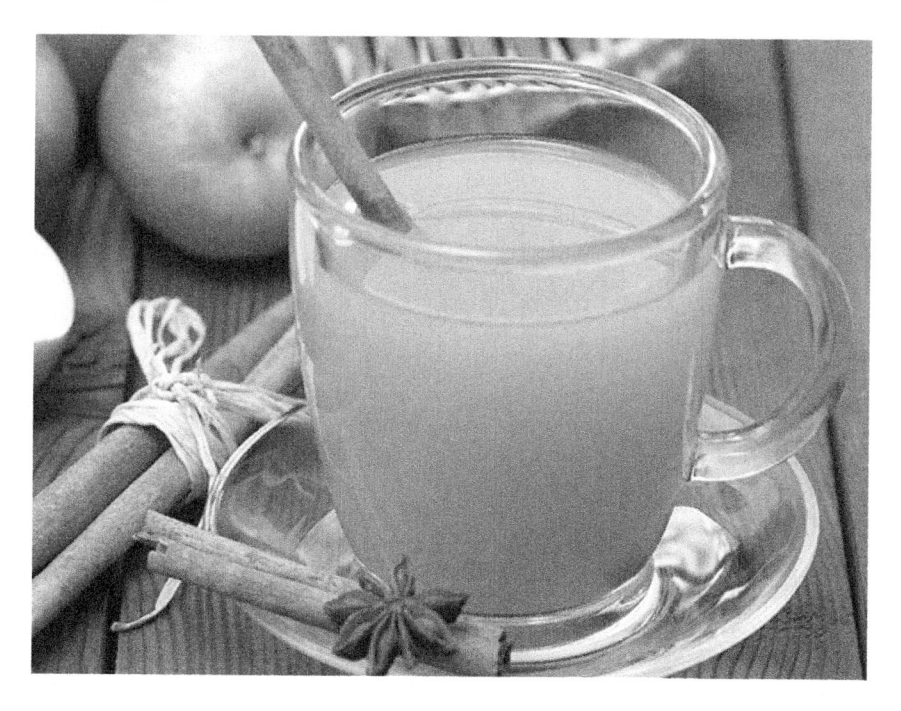

Ingredients:

- 4-6 apples, juiced (will make about 4 cups)
- 4 whole cloves
- 4 whole cinnamon sticks
- 4 whole cardamom pods
- 1-inch piece ginger
- ½ teaspoon lemon zest
- small orange, thin slices

Instructions:

1. Wash apples, then chop and prepare to suit your juicer.
2. Juice apples and transfer juice to a medium saucepan.
3. Add cloves, cinnamon, cardamom, ginger and lemon zest.
4. Cover and warm on low-medium for 25 minutes. Don't bring to a boil.
5. Add orange slices to the mixture in the last 5 minutes.
6. Strain the mixture into a heat-safe container or serve in your favorite mugs.

Prep Time: 35 min

Servings: 4-6

Poached Pear Smoothie

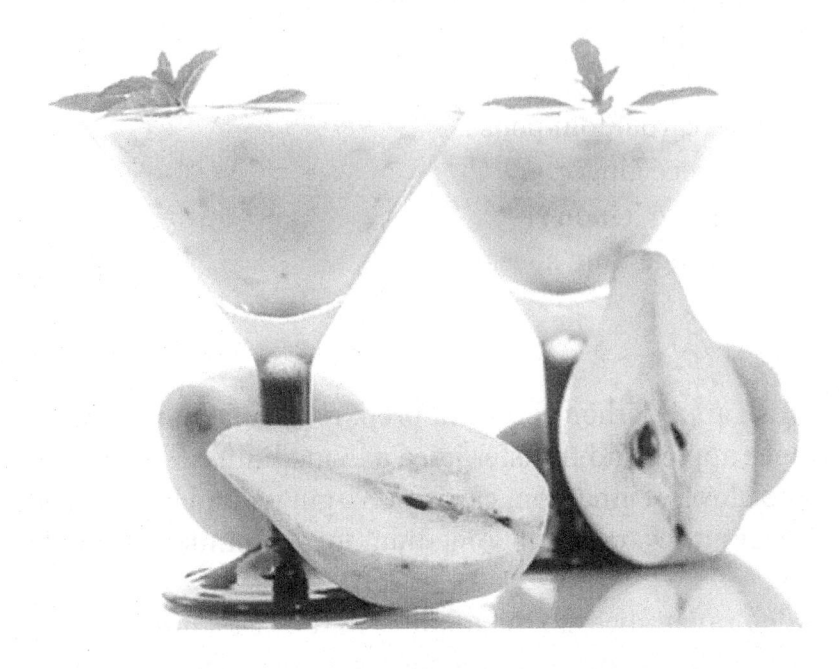

Ingredients:

- pear
- 1 ½ cup of almond milk
- ¼ tsp of ground cinnamon
- Pinch of nutmeg
- 1-2 dates (pitted)
- 1 scoop natural or vanilla protein powder (optional)
- 1 tsp of chia seeds (optional)

Instructions:

1. Wash and chop the pear into bite-sized pieces.
2. In a saucepan add chopped pear, almond milk, cinnamon, and nutmeg, simmer over medium heat for 5 to 7 minutes or until pear chunks are soft.
3. Add the pear mixture and remaining ingredients into a blender (slightly cooled for a glass blender) and blend.
4. Add a little pinch of nutmeg and cinnamon. Serve in a large mug or a heat-safe glass.

Prep Time: 10 min

Servings: 1-2

Gingerbread Cookie Smoothie

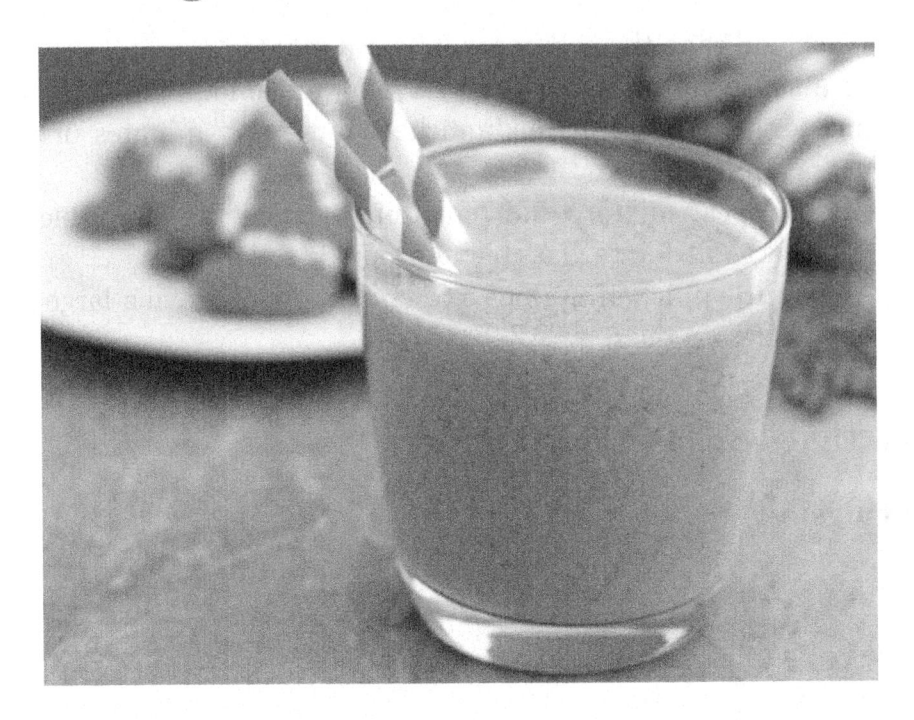

Ingredients:

- cup non-dairy milk (works great with this Oat Milk Recipe)
- 1 tablespoon almond butter (or your favorite nut/seed butter)
- 1 tablespoon blackstrap molasses
- 1 teaspoon vanilla extract
- 1/2 banana, peeled
- 1 teaspoon ground cinnamon
- 1/2 teaspoon fresh ground ginger
- 1/4 teaspoon nutmeg
- 1/8 teaspoon ground cloves

Instructions:

1. Add the ingredients to a high-powered blender and blend until smooth and creamy.
2. Transfer the mixture to a small saucepan set on medium heat and bring to a simmer. If the smoothie looks too thick, add an extra splash of non-dairy milk until desired consistency is reached.
3. When your smoothie reaches your preferred temperature, transfer it to a heat-safe glass or mug and enjoy!
4. If you want a little more indulgence, top it with some vegan whipped cream and cinnamon.

Prep Time: 10 min

Servings: 1-2

Cold Fighting Green Smoothie

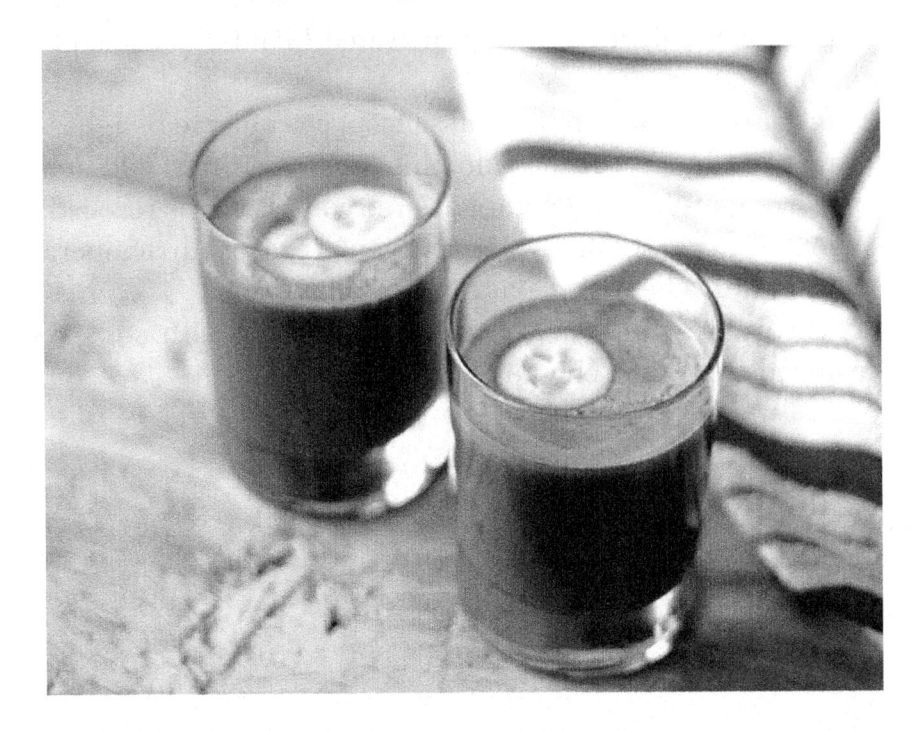

Ingredients:

- cup coconut water
- 1/4 cucumber
- tbsp live cultures natural yogurt
- 1/2 banana
- kiwis
- handfuls of spinach
- 1/4 tsp spirulina
- 10 drops Echinacea

Instructions:

4. Peel the kiwi, wash the cucumber and cut them into cubes.
5. Add all ingredients to the blender and mix until the ingredients are smooth.
6. Enjoy!!

Prep Time: 5 min

Servings: 1

Summer Refreshing Smoothies

This hydrating summer juices are refreshing, seasonal and will help you stay hydrated and feeling energized even on the hottest of days.

Try refreshing summer juices as a meal or snack replacement, to keep you cool and hydrated.

The Hydration Smoothie

Contains an awesome amount of phytonutrients from the watermelon and pineapple.

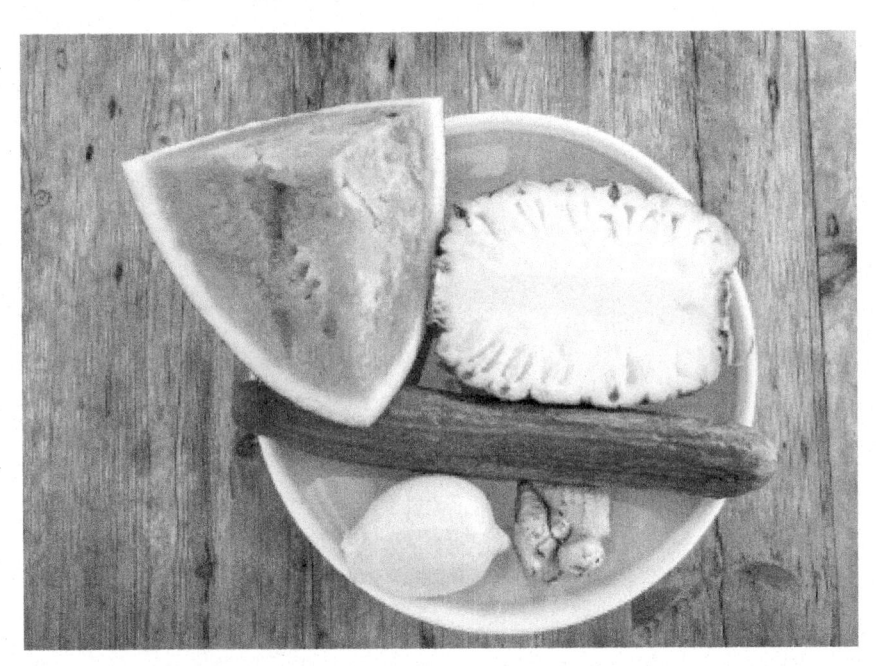

Ingredients:

- 1/2 pineapple
- 1/4 watermelon
- cucumber
- 1 lemon
- 1 inch (2.5 cm) piece of fresh ginger

Instructions:

1. Peel pineapple and lemon.
2. Wash all produce well.
3. Add all ingredients through juicer and enjoy!

Prep Time: 5 min

Servings: 2

Refreshing Coconut Lime Smoothie

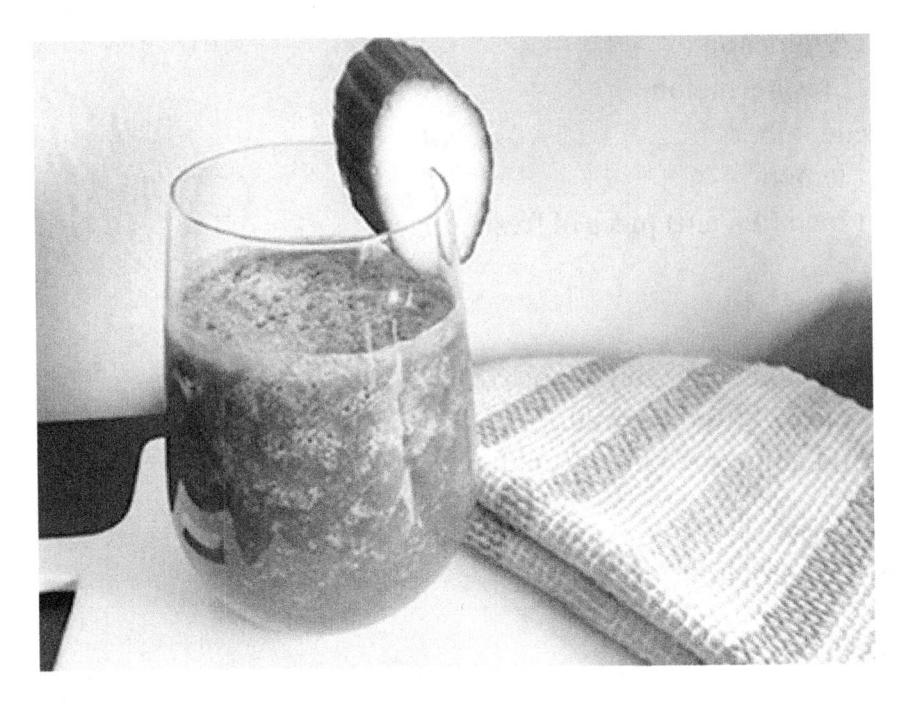

Ingredients:

- cup (250 ml) coconut water
- 1 pear, cored
- 1/3 cucumber
- 1 cup of spinach
- ½ lime, peeled
- 1 tsp coconut oil
- 1 handful of ice

Instructions:

1. Wash and prepare ingredients .
2. Add ingredients to a blender and blend on high for 45-60 seconds until smooth.
3. Serve and enjoy!

Prep Time: 3 min

Servings: 1

Green Tea Juice

Do not know what to choose to freshen up in the hot season - juice or iced tea? Why not unite them? The content of vitamin C in lemon and pineapple helps to increase the antioxidant and anti-cancer properties of green tea. Green tea is also great for losing weight and controlling appetite.

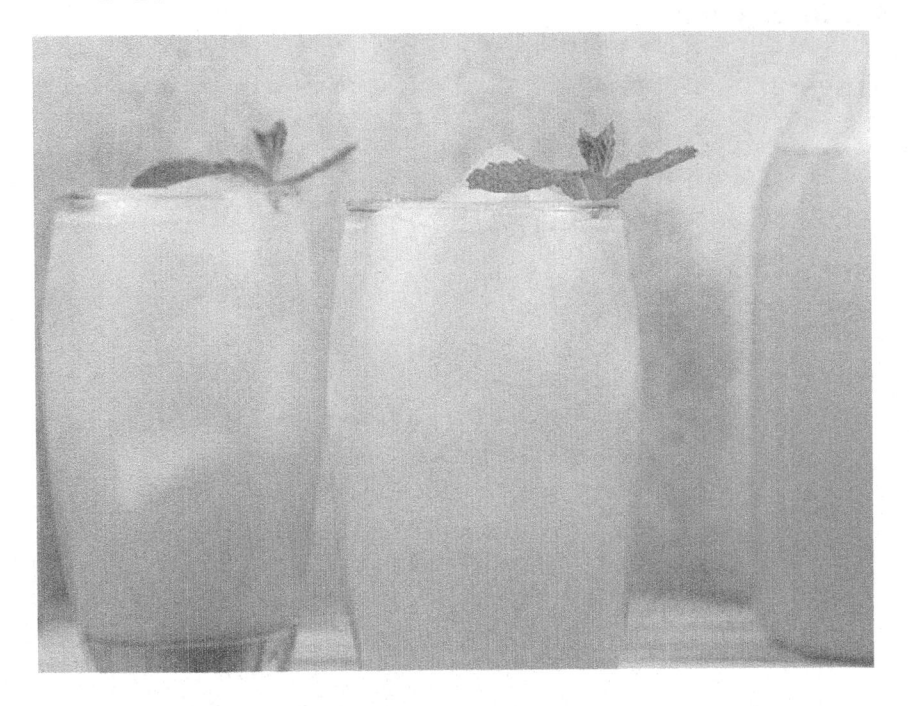

Ingredients:

- ¼ pineapple
- lemon
- 1 cup of cooled green tea

Instructions:

1. Peel the pineapple and scrub the lemon (peeling the lemon is optional).
2. Juice pineapple and lemon through a juicer.
3. Prepare the green tea and allow to cool.
4. Combine the pineapple and lemon juice with the green tea.
5. Add ice and enjoy!

Prep Time: 10 min

Servings: 1-2

Refreshing Watermelon Juice

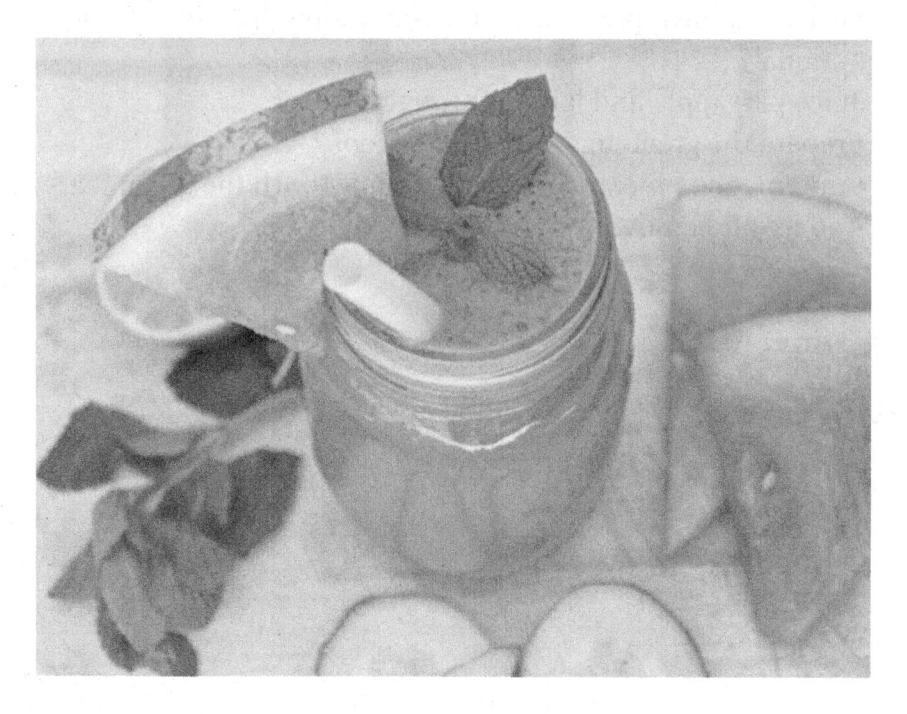

Ingredients:

- ¾ cup cut watermelon
- cucumber
- 4-5 leaves chard (rainbow or Swiss)
- ½ lime, peeled
- 3-4 sprigs mint

Instructions:

1. Wash and prepare ingredients.
2. Place everything in the blender and pulse until finely ground. The end result has to be smooth
3. Pour the juice into your favorite glass.
4. Enjoy!

Prep Time: 5 min

Servings: 1

Made in the USA
Monee, IL
25 January 2020